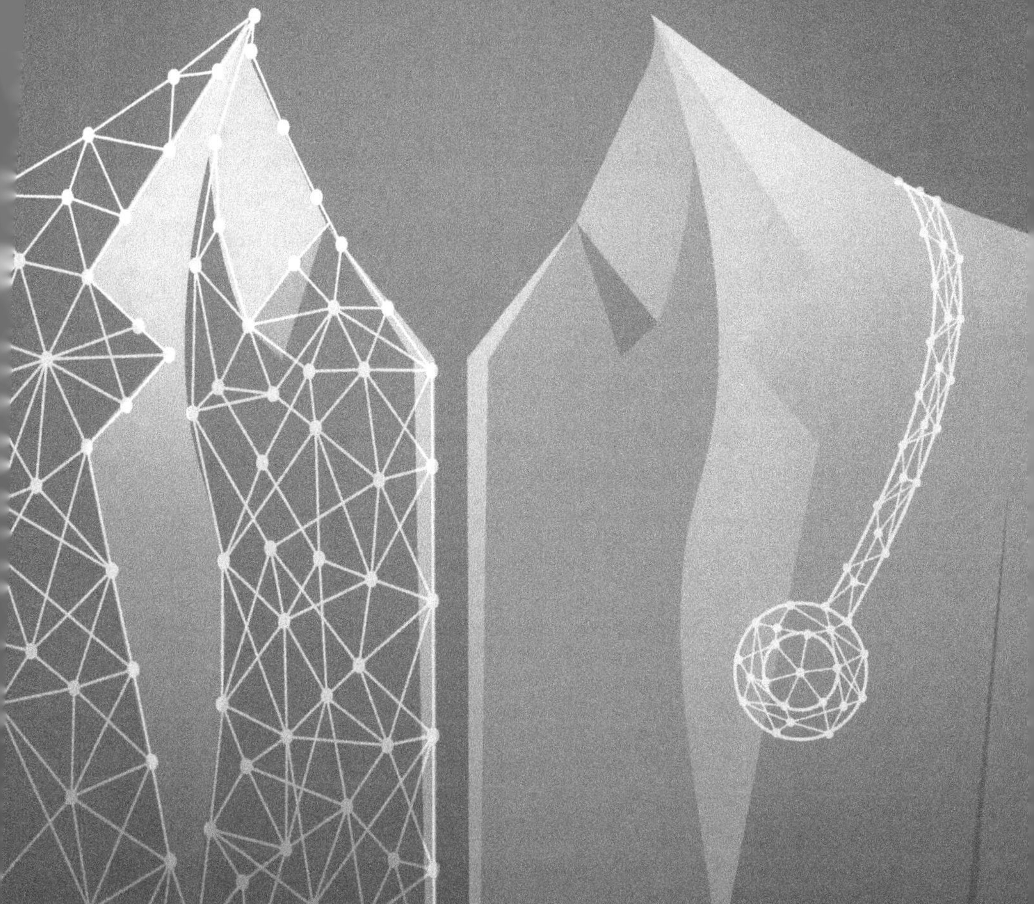

ESSAYS ON THE PRACTICE AND FUTURE OF MEDICINE

BECOMING TOMORROW'S DOCTOR

CHRISTOPHER M. CIRINO, DO, MPH

I dedicate this book to my parents,
Virginia and Antonio Cirino,
who planted the seed for my journey to becoming a doctor
through their words of encouragement and support.

I also dedicate this book to my children,
Gianluca, Sebastiano, and Enzo:
follow your dreams, and may the reality
that manifests be even better.

ISBN: 979-8-9869040-0-9 (hardcover)
ISBN: 979-8-9869040-1-6 (paperback)
ISBN: 979-8-9869040-2-3 (ebook)

Printed in the United States of America

10 9 8 7 6 5 4 3 2 1

ESSAYS ON THE PRACTICE AND FUTURE OF MEDICINE

BECOMING TOMORROW'S DOCTOR

CHRISTOPHER M. CIRINO, DO, MPH

Contents

The Hippocratic Oath[1]

I swear by Apollo Healer, by Asclepius, by Hygiea, by Panacea, and by all the gods and goddesses, making them my witnesses, that I will carry out, according to my ability and judgment, this oath and this indenture.

To hold my teacher in this art equal to my own parents; to make him partner in my livelihood; when he is in need of money to share mine with him; to consider his family as my own brothers, and to teach them this art, if they want to learn it, without fee or indenture; to impart precept, oral instruction, and all other instruction to my own sons, the sons of my teacher, and to indentured pupils who have taken the Healer's oath, but to nobody else.

I will use those dietary regimens which will benefit my patients according to my greatest ability and judgment, and I will do no harm or injustice to them. Neither will I administer a poison to anybody when asked to do so, nor will I suggest such a course. Similarly, I will not give to a woman a pessary to cause abortion. But I will keep pure and holy both my life and my art. I will not use the knife, not even, verily, on sufferers from stone, but I will give place to such as are craftsmen therein.

Into whatsoever houses I enter, I will enter to help the sick, and I will abstain from all intentional wrong-doing and harm, especially from abusing the bodies of man or woman, bond or free. And whatsoever I shall see or hear in the course of my profession, as well as outside my profession in my intercourse with men, if it be what should not be published abroad, I will never divulge, holding such things to be holy secrets.

Now if I carry out this oath, and break it not, may I gain forever reputation among all men for my life and for my art; but if I break it and forswear myself, may the opposite befall me.

The Osteopathic Oath

I do hereby affirm my loyalty to the profession I am about to enter. I will be mindful always of my great responsibility to preserve the health and the life of my patients, to retain their confidence and respect both as a physician and a friend who will guard their secrets with scrupulous honor and fidelity, to perform faithfully my professional duties, to employ only those recognized methods of treatment consistent with good judgment and with my skill and ability, keeping in mind always nature's laws and the body's inherent capacity for recovery.

I will be ever vigilant in aiding in the general welfare of the community, sustaining its laws and institutions, not engaging in those practices which will in any way bring shame or discredit upon myself or my profession. I will give no drugs for deadly purposes to any person, though it be asked of me.

I will endeavor to work in accord with my colleagues in a spirit of progressive cooperation and never by word or by act cast imputations upon them or their rightful practices.

I will look with respect and esteem upon all those who have taught me my art. To my college I will be loyal and strive always for its best interests and for the interests of the students who will come after me. I will be ever alerted to further the application of basic biologic truths to the healing arts and to develop the principles of osteopathy which were first enunciated by Andrew Taylor Still.

Preface

The graduation ceremony for medical school is a memorable milestone for students. The new graduates recite the Hippocratic and Osteopathic oaths as a rite of passage— marking their transition from student to doctor. Even in the modern era of medicine, these messages resonate. Medicine is as much a profession as it is a calling. It asks its doctors to use their knowledge and decision-making gained in training as tools to serve others. They make this pledge to their patients, colleagues, and community.

I have tremendous gratitude for the profession of medicine. I still find it hard to believe that I began my journey more than twenty-five years ago. In many ways, the goal of a fulfilling career was enough incentive to persevere through the hurdles along the way. The profession offers me the privilege of caring for others. Equally, it inspires me with a voracious curiosity about the human experience.

My attending physicians and other mentors gave plenty of sound advice during training. These experiences enhanced my practice, balancing my naïve idealism with healthy doses of reality. Similarly, I thought it was the right time to share my experiences with students and anyone curious about healthcare.

Since the outset of the pandemic, pre-health and medical students have faced disruptions in clinical rotations and shadowing opportunities. One of my jobs during the pandemic was to communicate with hospitals, practice groups, and doctors to find preceptors for medical students. Many of them went months without direct patient exposure. It was frustrating to hear similar statements from the clinics and hospitals I called: "We are not yet ready to take students for rotations. Check back with us in the next six months." Although online conferencing and coursework provided education and facilitated social distancing, the loss of direct observation has had ramifications. This book provides a format for delivering crucial aspects of a physician's career to this audience.

The writing consists of a collection of essays and case anecdotes woven together to give a perspective on the practice of medicine. For consistency, I use "physician" and "doctor." However, the subject matter applies to all healthcare providers, including nurses, physician assistants, nurse practitioners, and others in the healing arts.

The cases in this book represent the histories of individuals I have had the privilege of being a physician and ally. I omitted specifics to protect the identity of the patients and allow the reader to focus on the instruction of the narratives. The information appears to fall neatly into specific chapters, but the learning opportunities every patient provides a doctor cut across many areas. For my patients, I provided health and treatment advice and was available for a handhold or a hug. The topics form a patchwork of one physician's career, which has matured and transformed.

My practice has been one of ongoing learning and challenges. I can tell you that I am fascinated with how much we have discovered about the human condition and curious about how the physician's role will evolve. High school and college students contemplating careers in medicine will see it practiced much differently than today. They will become tomorrow's doctors and enter a field where technology fuels a new understanding of health. While they will embrace the future, they must not abandon the essential skills that have benefited both doctor and patient since the dawn of the profession: active listening, communication, and empathy.

I am forever grateful to my mentors and colleagues. They have shown me the promise of a fulfilling medical career and continue to demonstrate a physician's potential by leading through their compassionate example. I am also indebted to my patients, who have entrusted me with their deepest concerns and whom I've had the privilege to support during vulnerable times.

CHAPTER ONE

On Becoming a Physician: My Journey

The dedicated doctor knows that [they] must be both scientist and humanitarian. [Their] most agonizing decisions lie in the field of human relations.
-David B. Allman

Key Points

• Students preparing for medical school benefit from more than grade point averages, Medical College Admissions Test (MCAT) scores, and shadowing quotas. Self-esteem, adaptability, and stability offer protection from the rigors of medical school and practice.

• Within the US, there are two options for medical school training: Allopathic and Osteopathic medicine.

• Osteopathic medicine developed as an alternative to medical practices in the era of its inception. It emphasizes the body's healing ability and the importance of understanding the interplay of the body's structure and function.

What does it take to get into medical school?

That is a question many students ask as they prepare to apply for medical school. The steps to entering this professional training are among the most rigorous for any field of study. In 2021, there were a total of 62,443 applicants to 155 accredited MD-granting schools and 37 Osteopathic medical schools in the US, and the overall acceptance rate into any medical school was 41% (AAMC, 2021.) However, for the top 100 US News ranked medical schools, the average acceptance rate dropped to 6.3%. And schools like Florida State University, Stanford, New York University, and George Washington University have acceptance rates below 3% (Kerr, 2021).

Students' typical concerns about medical school admissions include MCAT scores, grade point averages (GPA), and extra-curricular activities, such as clinical exposure, volunteer opportunities, and research. Many schools factor in MCAT scores more strongly because they are a way to compare applicants objectively. Indeed lower MCAT and GPA scores predict the probability that a student will have trouble in medical school (Desy, 2021). In a meta-analysis of twenty-three studies, MCAT scores showed a small to medium predictive validity on medical school and clinical performance (Tyrone, 2007).

However, some traits are more critical than ranking a candidate based on test scores and grades. Life skills such as self-esteem, adaptability, and stability are beneficial in preparing one for intensive training and a service career. Individuals with a more stable childhood and adolescence have a lower likelihood of marital problems and drug dependence as physicians (Vaillant, 1972).

While admission to medical school has recently favored a more diverse, holistic applicant pool, several key attributes stand out. The Association of American Medical Colleges (AAMC) identifies fifteen core competencies listed in four categories: interpersonal, intrapersonal, reasoning, and science (AAMC website). This book addresses several of these competencies. Keep in mind that while you ask yourself what medical schools look for, think about what life skills you can develop to approach a career in medicine with support and resilience.

Core Competencies for Entering Medical Students (AAMC)

Interpersonal Competences

- Service Orientation
- Social Skills
- Cultural Competence
- Teamwork
- Oral Communication

Intrapersonal Competencies

- Ethical Responsibility to Self and Others
- Reliability and Dependability
- Resilience and Adaptability
- Capacity for Improvement

Thinking and Reasoning Competencies

- Critical Thinking
- Quantitative Reasoning
- Scientific Inquiry
- Written Communication

Science Competencies

- Living Systems
- Human Behavior

What is the Difference Between a D.O. and a M.D.?

In the United States, there are two types of medical schools that provide training to become a doctor: Osteopathic Medicine and Allopathic Medicine; the schools offer degrees in Doctor of Osteopathic Medicine (D.O.) or Medical Doctor (M.D.), respectively. As of 2021, there were 1,062,205 physicians practicing in the United States (Michas, 2021). Of the total, almost 135,000 are osteopathic physicians (AOA, 2021). Currently, 1 in 4 US medical students attends an osteopathic medical school.

Allopathic Medicine is a general term, representing what people consider modern, Western medicine. Technology and research methods drive the advancements in medicine. Currently, applicants can choose among 152 US MD schools. There are 133 accredited specialty and subspecialty residency programs by the Accreditation Council of Graduate Medical Education (ACGME). Allopathic training programs provide their students and residents with an extensive educational opportunity, clinical research, and subspecialty coverage.

Andrew Taylor Still founded the first Osteopathic medical school in Kirksville, Missouri in 1892. Today, there are 38 accredited osteopathic medical schools in 59 locations in the United States (AACOM). In addition to the traditional medical school curriculum, osteopathic students receive at least 200 hours of training in palpatory skills and osteopathic manipulative medicine (OMM). Osteopathic programs are known for a strong commitment to primary care.

The main tenets of Osteopathic Medicine approved by the American Osteopathic Association (AOA) House of Delegates are the following statements:

- The body is a unit; the person is a unit of body, mind, and spirit.
- The body is capable of self-regulation, self-healing, and health maintenance.
- Structure and function are reciprocally interrelated.
- Rational treatment is based upon an understanding of the basic principles of body unity, self-regulation, and the interrelationship of structure and function.

The two disciplines have converged in the last few decades, including the formation of a uniform system of graduate medical education in 2021.

My Journey

I did not come from a pedigree of doctors. My brother and I were the first two in the family. My parents significantly influenced my career choice but in different ways.

My father emigrated to the United States, lured by the American Dream. He grew up in poverty in a small village in southern Italy, where nothing came easily— not even education. He frequently spoke of his struggles to complete his studies, including lack of funding, long walks during cold winters to a school in the closest city, and gaining the support of a professor, who provided him with the required books that he could not afford.

My father's trip to the United States began as a visit with relatives but became the start of his family when he met and married my mother after a few dates. In five years, our family was complete, and he was fortunate to find a stable, manual job to provide for us. Naturally, his motivations extended to his children. My dad thought that if his children could be doctors, they would not have the poverty he faced growing up. In Italy, being a doctor is among the most respected professions.

As a child, I often heard my parents tell me that I should be a doctor. Later as a teenager, they would remind me that I had always wanted to be a doctor. I admit I felt some pressure with my career somehow being predetermined. Somewhere in between, I must have agreed with them. I did enjoy school, maintained good grades, and liked science and mathematics. However, neither they nor I knew what becoming a physician entailed.

My childhood experiences fueled my interest in science and, more specifically, microbiology, the field I chose for my college major and medical training. It was fascinating to see a new world under a microscope I received one childhood Christmas. I would sometimes place saliva or a skin sample on a slide to see the sheets of cells. I imagined the scientists who discovered microbes in pond water using the prototypical microscopes they made from lenses. They were like explorers in a new world.

My mother completed nursing school while I was a teenager. I felt a sense of pride and respect for my mother as she worked toward her career goals. My brothers and I would listen to her discuss diseases with her classmates while studying together. I was intrigued by her textbooks, which had photos of patients with exotic infections. Those books and others were a pathway toward clarifying the unknown.

In the late 1970s, the world faced an uncertain pandemic with increasing reports of a condition that led to immune deficiency. People with Acquired Immunodeficiency Syndrome (AIDS) were contracting rare infections and cancers, and the most significant risk groups were men-who-have-sex-with-men, hemophiliacs, and people who abused intravenous drugs. In 1983, virologists Luc Montagnier and Françoise Barré-Sinoussi isolated what later became known as the Human Immunodeficiency Virus (HIV) (Barré-Sinoussi, 1983). In 1984, virologist Gallo isolated the virus from a lymph node of someone with AIDS and confirmed it to be a retrovirus (Gallo, 2003). As I listened to the news reports on television, I became fascinated by infectious diseases. The logic of uncovering a greater understanding of life's mysteries appealed to me.

In college, I participated in research activities, had opportunities to instruct other students, and even taught children in primary schools about microbiology. Working with a faculty advisor, I prepared a research project that included feeding mice specific amino-acid deficient diets and injecting them with leukemia cells. The goal was to determine the effects of diet on the immune system. Although the results were not compelling, the process exposed me to experimental trials. All these experiences galvanized my interests in science and teaching. But how did this translate to becoming a doctor?

The time came to apply to medical schools. I attended an informational session on Osteopathic medicine at my college. I learned about Osteopathy's founding father, Andrew Taylor (A.T.) Still, and the medical practices standard during his lifetime (1828-1917) (Tan, 2007). Methods such as bloodletting, arsenic, whiskey, and opium were treatments in that era. A.T. Still faced hardships, including losing three children to meningitis and his first wife to childbirth. These tragedies fueled him to look for answers beyond those that medicine at that time could offer. He began studying the human body.

A.T. Still contended that "the job of a physician is to find health. Anybody can find disease." Along with this maxim, he supported the notion that the body functioned as a unified organism with an innate ability to heal, hearkening back to the teachings of Hippocrates and the concept of physis. These healing constructs continue to be a source of intrigue for me today.

While preparing the personal statement for my medical school application, I pondered the question that I started this chapter with: do I have what it takes to be a doctor? Not everyone thought I did. My college microbiology professor advised me that I was more suited for graduate school— that I was better with things than with people. Maybe he's right, I remember thinking. However, after being a "lab rat" for a few years and spending occasional weekends and evenings isolated in a lab, I did not see myself doing something similar for a career. I valued the personal, human connection that comes with being a doctor.

Unfortunately, I was unsure my MCAT scores would be high enough to be accepted into medical school. And it was not because I did not study for them. I read chapters out of bulky textbooks every day for several months, but I did not have access to test questions. Later, I realized that going through test questions and using them to fine-tune knowledge gaps was a better way to prepare for the multiple standardized exams that students take. A good night's rest and a distraction-free environment on test day are equally crucial.

The other question that I asked was whether I wanted to become a doctor. At twenty-one, I had difficulty imagining a seven-year commitment to medical education and residency training. After some soul-searching, I decided to follow through with the applications. My primary fascination growing up was understanding how the body functions and heals itself. If I wanted to pursue research later, I would not burn any bridges by becoming a doctor. Osteopathic medicine offered me focused time to consider the integral role of our bodies in health. Both Osteopathic and Allopathic schools contacted me for admission. Intrigued by the teachings of A.T. Still, I chose the former and prepared myself for medical education at the Ohio University College of Osteopathic Medicine.

Medical school was the most exciting and expansive educational experience in my life. I selected the Problem-Based Learning (PBL) track that my medical school had launched the year of my enrollment. The smaller faculty-to-student ratio, the case-based format, students functioning as their instructors, and the independent learning were appealing. I thought this program could serve as an apprenticeship in medicine and prepare me for lifelong learning. Studies support that PBL does offer medical students some advantages in social and cognitive dimensions, such as coping with uncertainty, communication skills, and self-directed study (Koh, 2008.) These are valuable skills for future doctors.

I was ready to start as an attending physician after four years of medical school, a year of rotating internship, three years of residency, and two years of fellowship. And the learning continues. I acquired knowledge about diseases during my formative years but would spend the rest of my career understanding health.

The Journey of Tomorrow's Doctor

Becoming a doctor begins with gaining a foundation of knowledge and decision-making. Doctors strive to provide patients with an accurate diagnosis using limited information. Training prepares doctors to make better predictions, even when conditions are still developing. Doctors also learn to implement the many tools of the trade, including stethoscopes, otoscopes, and technology. Research and discovery expand their ability to more effectively diagnosis and treat conditions.

We are at a turning point in healthcare. We have witnessed the shift from healthcare to "sick care," even as we gain tremendous insight into science and technology. As chronic diseases grow in prevalence, the systems used yesterday and today must evolve to encourage the capacity of individuals to heal themselves. The restoration of health remains an invitation and opportunity for every patient who develops a disease brought on by behaviors. Doctors cannot prescribe pills to change behaviors.

Doctors will have to redefine their role in an ever-changing environment to avoid becoming technicians. While technology will facilitate medical care, it will not replace the need for human connection. The doctor-patient relationship might look different in the future, but compassionate care continues to be integral to optimal healthcare. The bridge that empathy builds between the two strengthens care and is transformative. It offers an avenue to address behaviors. The ability of a therapeutic relationship to activate the body's healing through behavior change is nothing short of a miracle. We cannot abandon the doctor-patient relationship as we embrace the future of medicine.

As healthcare evolves, we must support the elements that distinguish quality, growth-promoting doctor-patient alliances over today's band-aid, subsistence practices. Tomorrow's doctors must prepare themselves for innovative technology yet remain mindful of the importance of doctor-patient connection and collaboration. These are the quintessential ingredients to quality and awakened healthcare.

About the Book

The chapters in this book cover crucial elements for future doctors. The primary intended audience is the student contemplating the field of medicine. I prepared the text to include material that I would have found helpful as a pre-medical student. Current and future doctors, healthcare workers, and developers of health system models will also find this content informative and relevant to their work.

The perspectives come from one individual – inescapably biased by being white and male – and are offered with the disclaimer that they are not representative of every student's unique path. Diversity and inclusion are beneficial and necessary in healthcare. I want to acknowledge the hurdles that many women and minority students still face. Sexual prejudice, and racial and gender bias in medicine continue to be obstacles for practicing physicians. They must endure salary disparities, microaggressions, and increased burnout and depression rates (Ly, 2016; Dudley, 2022). Although the themes covered in this book are generalizable, I encourage readers to review other materials to supplement their understanding.

I hope this book will serve you, whether you would like to become a doctor, are currently in med school, or are simply curious about the journey. The practice of medicine is like an unfinished symphony. Tomorrow's doctors and other healthcare workers will shape the trajectory of the next opus. What promises does the future of medicine hold for the world?

CHAPTER 2

The Evolution of the Modern Health Paradigm

All is darkness and confusion, vague theory, and vain speculation. Is it a fungus, an insect, a miasm, an electrical disturbance, a deficiency of ozone, a morbid off-scouring from the intestinal canal? We know nothing; we are at sea in a whirlpool of conjecture.
—T. Wakley, Founder of *The Lancet.* Editorial on Cholera. *The Lancet* II, 393, 1853

Key Points

- Our senses predict, interpret, and project our reality.
- A physician cultivates sensory skills to improve the prediction of a patient's illness.
- Consciousness is a learned behavior where the brain tests hypotheses, developed from past experiences, as it interacts with the world.
- The health paradigm shapes the perspectives in which people view health and disease. As we gain insight into the mechanisms of the body, we continue to refine the paradigm.

Introduction: Practicing Medicine

In the United States, students attend four years of medical school after college and then train in a residency program for another three to seven years. These formative years become an amalgam of training, unique for everyone. As physicians-in-training progress through these stages and acquire more experience, they gain greater responsibility in each patient's care and refine their interpretative and decision-making skills.

Lifelong learning makes *practicing* medicine an apt term. As students recall lessons, errors, and exceptions, they calibrate their ability to interpret, intuit, and predict. They develop pattern recognition skills and apply shorthand rules to assess patients. The more students and residents practice, the better prepared they will be. The learning never stops. It only adapts and develops, as does a career in medicine.

Nevertheless, a solid background in basic and clinical sciences is not enough to be a successful doctor. Newer technologies, like advanced radiology, integrated electronic medical records, and artificial intelligence, may enhance but cannot replace the physician's role. The practice of medicine lives at the interface of human-to-human interaction.

Medical Training and the Five Senses

The profession of doctor dates back more than 25,000 years. Early physicians had few tools to assist them. Sharpening the five senses became an integral part of training.[2] They closely listened to patients explain what was wrong with them. Physicians used their hands to identify fluid around the lungs, joint swelling, or an enlarged liver or spleen with palpation (touch) and percussion (tapping) skills. Their eyes scanned the skin for clues of systemic disease or discerned changes in urine or stool. They relied on smell and even taste to detect any signs of illness, such as checking urine for findings suggestive of diabetes.

Today physicians still undergo intensive training to develop sensory skills and expand their knowledge base. The difference between a beginning student and a finishing resident is like a novice artist and an experienced artist painting an image of a mountain on a canvas. The beginner's art may include the right colors, but it lacks details and accurate dimensions. An artist who has fine-tuned their skills over many years captures a more realistic image. Similarly, doctors develop methods to interpret reality better.

Understanding the spoken word and listening beyond hearing requires training. Doctors must learn how to communicate and determine the contextual meaning of the words. During a clinical visit, a patient recounts their experiences. They select words to describe the symptoms and make assumptions based on their perceptions. The doctor's interpretation of the story also relies on assumptions, entangling both narratives in bias. The actual, emerging cause of a condition may become blurred.

Obtaining a thorough record of a patient's illness is crucial. The omission of essential information may lead a doctor down the wrong path. Without asking the right questions, a doctor misses a broader spectrum of possibilities. They may conclude that anyone who reports coughing and fever has pneumonia. However, someone returning from the tropics with a cough, fever, and lung changes may have many diseases, including Katayama syndrome, tuberculosis, or leptospirosis. The information lies in waiting for the doctor to ask.

Assessments Draw from the Past

We use our knowledge and experience to understand the world around us. When these are limited, we attempt to interpret something using what we know. But our conclusions are often oversimplified and prone to error, primarily when we evaluate the unfamiliar.

Imagine you came from an island devoid of technology. How would you describe a car with no prior knowledge of it? You might notice its shape is like a canoe frame, or that it sounds like an animal when the motor revs up, or the headlights look like large torches. However, none of these descriptions capture what a car is. How would your observations differ if you were an experienced car mechanic?

A student takes a similar journey in becoming a physician. They improve their skills to assess and determine the cause of a patient's concerns. People can only gain perspective by dynamically observing and interacting with a person, situation, or object. The senses enable the brain to design an experience of reality, and the memory gives it a context.

Health Paradigms Drive Perspectives

Humans have grappled through time with how to relate to health and the body's inner workings. An understanding of health requires a lens, or *paradigm*, through which to interpret it. The term paradigm relates to a collective viewpoint that guides the development of theories in a particular field (Heikkinen, 2000). A health paradigm attempts to explain the forces that occur in the body. Paradigm shifts have occurred throughout history when more accurate theories replaced or clarified less accurate ones. These shifts often lead to both destructive and constructive changes in scientific thought. The objective is to reach an accord between theory and fact (Kuhn, 1962).

Often, a paradigm shift occurs gradually and follows the *diffusion of innovation* mechanics, a social phenomenon that describes how a discovery or technology spreads to the public (**Figure 1**) (Dearing,

2018.) The early adopters of a new health paradigm are medical and scientific community members. They assess the validity, benefits, and risks of adopting a new theory. Scientists weigh the theory's importance, timeliness, and even the innovator's influence (Dearing, 2018). Sometimes, presenting a more practical idea does not guarantee that people will adopt it.

A theory with multiple anomalies is inaccurate and of limited value. Scientists refine a theory by testing hypotheses and collecting evidence to refute or support it. Rarely a finding alters the fundamental principles of the theory. A scientist who breaks away from a majority viewpoint risks rejection or loss of confidence in the scientific community. However, scientific rigor and technology facilitate a paradigm shift by strengthening evidence. You will see how the microscope led to a departure from old paradigms.

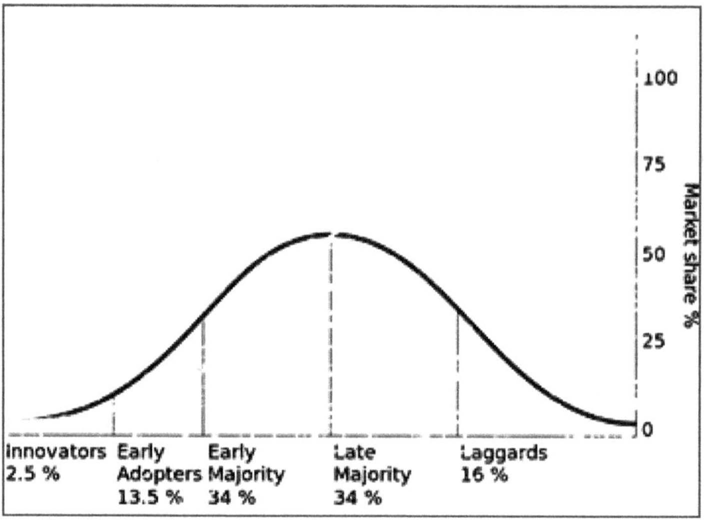

Figure 1: Diffusion of Innovation. Source: Wikimedia Commons.

The Past as Prologue: Early Health Paradigms

Doctors of the past applied less dependable health models than doctors do today. Some early theories included astrology, humorism, and miasmas. Imagine having to factor in the positions of the heavenly bodies before an emergency surgery today. It is valuable to discuss some of these, underscoring that they were driven by natural observations and narratives attempting to explain them. Aspiring doctors gain a framework to evaluate current and emerging paradigms presented at the end of the chapter.

The Four Humors

The theory of the four humors, or humorism, became prevalent after the Greeks Empedocles (494-434 B.C.E) and Hippocrates (460-375 B.C.E) expanded on earlier Egyptian and Mesopotamian teachings. Empedocles espoused that all substances in the universe, including the body, consisted of air, fire, water, and earth. The theory tied these elements to four bodily substances, or *humors*: yellow bile, blood, phlegm, and black bile. According to the theory, health exists when they are in harmony, while illness occurs from disharmony (Lagay, 2002).

In the first century AD, the Greek surgeon Galen (129-216 AD) interrogated nature, further codifying the theory. "Nature does nothing in vain," he declared (Dunn, 2003). He gained greater insight of it by conducting animal dissections and vivisections (West, 2014). Additionally, Galen developed the notion that an imbalance in the four humors contributed to various personality types or temperaments, including sanguine, melancholic, phlegmatic, and choleric (Flaskerud, 2012).

Humorism became the paradigm to frame health for the next eighteen centuries. In 1025, the Persian intellect Ibn Sina (980-1037 AD), or Avicenna wrote a pivotal medical text known as *The Canon of*

Medicine. Therein, he defined medicine as "the art whereby health is conserved and the art whereby it is restored after being lost." He also characterized the notion of illness, dividing it into three categories: temperament, structure, and loss of continuity. Avicenna claimed that someone is either healthy or ill, and that anything in-between is "health-in-decline." Although he added several concepts, woven into these were the themes of his predecessors, Galen, Aristotle, and Hippocrates (Heldreth, 2014). Some of his ideas influenced contemporary holistic theories of health.

Humorism was not a supernatural construct. Instead, it was formalized, albeit imprecisely, by the observation of bodily fluids and an elementary understanding of physiology. Attention to input also implied that doctors listened and learned about their patient's risk factors for disease. They asked questions about lifestyle choices, habits, and the influence of the environment the patient lived in and frequented (Legay, 2002).

Even through the 17th century, humorism was largely uncontested. The revelations in anatomy and physiology of Andreas Vesalius (1514-1564) and William Harvey (1578-1657) pioneered a movement toward a more accurate scientific method (West, 2014). However, there is often a gap between discovery and a shift to a universally accepted health paradigm.

Miasma Theory

Until the early twentieth century, infectious diseases were the leading cause of death. Even today, contagious diseases such as malaria, cholera, and tuberculosis significantly impact developing countries. The world has witnessed more than 6 million deaths since the outset of the COVID-19 pandemic in 2020. What makes these so dangerous is that they come from the environment and spread from person to person, which is hard to avoid.

An observation of a disease suddenly occurring and affecting many people made early doctors wonder whether the air was the culprit. Hippocrates (460-377 B.C.E.) posited the miasma theory to explain how the environment led to fatal epidemics in Greece during his lifetime (Kannadan, 2018). The idea held that miasmas, air tainted by rotting matter, were the source of disease. From Latin meaning "evil air," malaria earned its name because of the misconception that poisonous air was the cause, not mosquitoes as vectors.

Unlike humorism, miasma theory attributed disease to supernatural causes like evil spirits, ghosts, and gods. Our ancestors had no tools but their senses to ascribe reasons to observations. Early doctors endeavored to keep people healthy through a miasma lens by preventing air contamination. They supported clean air and sanitation measures to reduce pollution and the risk of infection.

The bubonic plague or Black Death was a formidable challenge to medieval Europe and responsible for the death of twenty-five million people— more than one-third of Europe (Glatter, 2021). Doctors like Charles de Lorme designed costumes to protect them from miasmas during the black plague in 17th-century Europe. These gowns were complete with a hat, goggles, and a bird mask filled with perfume and two small breathing holes (**Figure 2**) (Blakemore, 2020). Unfortunately, these outfits were no match for a tiny contagion transmitted by flea bites, not the air. Europe had a rat problem in the Middle Ages, and riding on the rodents were infected fleas that carried the bacteria that caused the plague. It took until 1894 for scientist Alexandre Yersin to identify the bacteria named after him, *Yersinia pestis* (Butler, 2014).

In 1854, epidemiologist John Snow's observations during a London cholera outbreak challenged the longstanding theory. Miasma-guided precautions had offered little help in curbing the infection rate (Kannadan, 2018). In his publication, Snow determined through empiricism that the common link in cholera infections was drinking from the same water source.

Snow concluded that cholera was a waterborne illness. Initially, these claims met resistance when local health authorities could not see past the limits of their paradigm (Greenhalgh, 2021). They regarded his conclusions as incorrect and laden with errors. In 1866, eight years after Snow's death and while London faced another cholera outbreak, it became undeniable that it was waterborne (Johnson, 2008).

Past theories depended on sensory observations and the brain's interpretations. They did not benefit from today's technological support. However, earlier beliefs were not wholly inaccurate. Infectious diseases such as tuberculosis and measles spread in an airborne manner but keeping the air fresh did not prevent them. When a theory no longer explains phenomena or offers protection, scientists must look further. It would take an essential innovation in the 1500s and more than three hundred years later to provide enough evidence to change the paradigm.

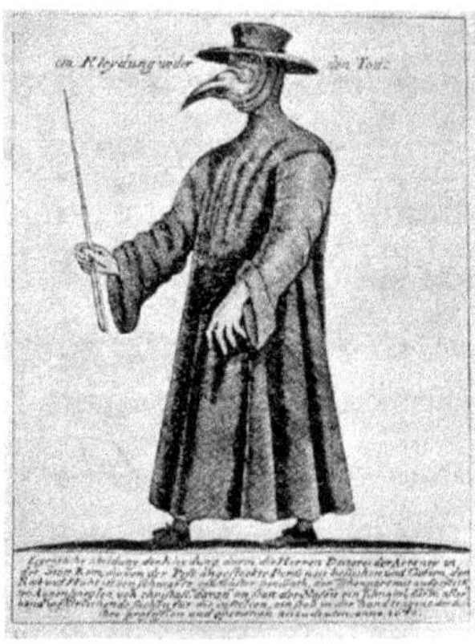

Figure 2: A Plague Doctor's Costume. Source Creative Commons

Paradigm Shift I: From Miasma to Germ Theory

Our brains narrate our vision of reality. Indeed, the impetus for redefining health was a lens that enhanced sight. In the late 16th century, the Janssens developed lenses for a handheld magnifying glass called a "microscope." Later iterations of microscopes over a century provided the resolution necessary for scientist Robert Hooke to define a new world in 1667 (Poppick, 2017).

Imagine being a scientist using a technology that completely discredited theories regarded as undisputable for millennia! The Germ theory states that microbes cause illnesses such as anthrax, cholera, malaria, and pneumonia. One could be a witness to these tiny organisms only with a microscope. At first, the scientific community regarded these pioneers as heretics.

Logic won over a faulty paradigm. German bacteriologist Robert Koch, the father of clinical microbiology, developed steps in classifying bacteria as causes of infections (**Table 1**) (Waler, 2021.) The postulates were not wholly accurate for all bacteria or viruses and prions. However, they represented a logical approach to confirming that specific germs cause illnesses. With such incontrovertible evidence, by the end of the 19th century, germ theory usurped miasma theory as the new standard.

Germ theory led to a new age of scientific discovery in infectious disease. By identifying the causes of infections, scientists developed methods to treat them with vaccinations and antibiotics. Prevention strategies could also be more fine-tuned. Health advancements came from the work of scientists and physicians like Robert Koch (Bacteriology), Louis Pasteur (Vaccinology, Pasteurization), Ignaz Semmelweis (Handwashing), Joseph Lister (Sanitation Measures), and Jonathan Snow (Epidemiology). As a result of these visionaries and improved public health measures, infectious diseases as a cause of death plummeted, and life expectancy increased.

Table 1. Koch's Postulates[3]
• The bacteria must be present in every case of the disease. • The bacteria must be isolated from the host with the disease and grown in pure culture. • The specific disease must be reproduced when a pure culture of the bacteria is inoculated into a healthy susceptible host. • The bacteria must be recoverable from the experimentally infected host.

The Biomedical Model and the Unanswered Burden of Chronic Diseases

Germ theory ushered in a new health paradigm— the **biomedical model**. The view held that evaluating the components of the body can provide a more complete understanding of health. Scientists could better comprehend diseases by looking at physical changes from a cellular level (Wade, 2004). The theory contributed to more empirical research methods, such as the randomized control trial—studies controlling variables to understand the effect of unknowns, including medications and other therapies.

The twentieth century marked an age of mass production of pharmaceuticals. Industries such as Bayer, originally a dye company in the 19th century, launched their first medicine, aspirin, in 1904. Bayer, along with other companies such as Squibb, Merck, and Pfizer, mass-produced antibiotics such as sulfonamides (1937), penicillin (1944), and Doxycycline (1953). In the 1960s and 1970s, drug companies turned to manage cancer, mental health, and chronic diseases. The first statin for high cholesterol was approved in 1987 and manufactured by Merck.

Chronic diseases such as heart disease, diabetes, and cancer have gained a stranglehold on an aging population. Today, almost half of U.S. Americans live with at least one chronic illness. More than two-thirds of deaths are attributable to chronic diseases, including cancer, hypertension, stroke, chronic obstructive pulmonary disease, and diabetes (Raghupathi, 2018). A burgeoning obesity epidemic coincides with these conditions.

The COVID-19 Pandemic Fueled Research and Understanding of Risk Factors

Outbreaks have a way of fueling scientific research, where curiosity meets necessity. The Severe Acute Respiratory Syndrome Coronavirus (SARS-CoV-2) and the disease it causes, Coronavirus disease 2019 (COVID-19), otherwise inexistent before December 2019, have become some of the most important research topics of all time. A PubMed literature search in April 2022 using the key terms "SARS-CoV-2" and "COVID-19" generated more than 150,000 and 240,000 articles, respectively, while the word "influenza," a disease described for centuries, had less than 150,000 results. While drafting this book, the Food and Drug Administration (FDA) approved three vaccines for COVID-19, and globally nine vaccines are approved (FDA site). Several became available within one year after the World Health Organization (WHO) declared that SARS-CoV-2 was a pandemic.

The WHO estimates that more than six million people have died from the pandemic (WHO site). The COVID-19 pandemic has been a wake-up call to the risks of chronic diseases, as infected individuals with obesity, diabetes, high blood pressure, and lung disease have had the worst outcomes. It also exposed health equity gaps in COVID-19 disease rates and outcomes, access to care, and vaccination rates, all of which were worse in poverty-stricken and

BIPOC communities (Black, Indigenous, and People of Color) (Andraska, 2021; Patel, 2020).

Paradigm Shift II: From the Biomedical Model Toward a Comprehensive View of Health

The biomedical model emerged on the backbone of discoveries that helped explain the body's components in greater detail and depended heavily on reductionism. Using trees as an example, it held that scientists could better understand them by looking at each of their components— the bark, leaves, root system, and branches. However, we lose information on how the systems communicate. We also run the risk of "not seeing the forest for the trees." In a paradigm that started primarily because of improved vision, the greater magnification has only accentuated the myopia of these views.

Could this be a time to improve the health paradigm? The healthcare and pharmaceutical industries have not addressed the current crisis. The rising prevalence of chronic diseases has cost lives and money. Health care is now primarily sick care, with approximately 78% of health spending on chronic conditions (Anderson, 2004). These diseases have one common link: behavior. Medications fall short of efficacy if underlying behaviors go unaddressed.

A more holistic approach provides a way to explain health as an interaction of multiple systems. In 1977, pathologist and psychiatrist George Engel referred to this broader focus as a **biopsychosocial model** (BPS) (Engel, 1977; Borrell-Carrió, 2004). A pathologist looks at tissue under a microscope to diagnose a condition like Crohn's disease or ulcerative colitis. A psychiatrist considers a patient's physical, social, and relational factors on brain health. Engel's unique skillset gave him a perspective to assess the brain's influences on physical findings and vice versa.

Instead of looking at the body and brain as isolated phenomena, the BPS model incorporates the dynamic interactions between the human body, psychology, and the social and environmental influences on health. Patients with chronic conditions are aware of how stress can be harmful to their health. A growing body of evidence has shown that stress impairs the immune system, exacerbates physical diseases like Crohn's disease, predisposes to cancer, and increases cardiovascular mortality (Yarieygi, 2017).

Health and behavior are intertwined and are adaptations to the environment. If we look at health from a molecular level, cells communicate locally and remotely with other cells. Neurotransmitters, hormones, and other molecules regulate gene expression and adaptative responses.

A pivotal study, the Adverse Childhood Experiences Study (ACES), showed the long-term effect of these responses on human health. There was a strong correlation between childhood trauma and the risk of developing chronic diseases as adults (Felitti, 1998).

Today's medical students spend 80% of their time learning biology, even when almost half of the premature deaths result from behavior (Schroeder, 2007). A more holistic approach to medical education and healthcare may offer a better way to address the nation's ailing health. For example, Trauma-Informed Primary Care (TIPC) represents a more comprehensive model on the interrelation between chronic conditions and adverse experiences (Roberts, 2019). Greater recognition of these themes and a compassionate communication style may improve a patient's health outcomes and the overall quality of care.

Today, scientific studies in fields like neuroscience and neurogenetics increase our clarity of how behavior interacts with the body's functions. In understanding the dynamic interaction between humans and their environment, a doctor can listen intently to how a person's narrative contributed to their health trajectory.

Implied is the possibility of modifying behavior, correcting disease, and releasing the body from dysfunction. With a foundation rooted in millennia of teachings, a new health paradigm is emerging.

The doctor of the future will give no medicine but will instruct his patient in the care of the human frame in diet and in the cause and prevention of disease.
Thomas Edison

CHAPTER 3

Transcending Bias in Clinical Decision-Making

Medicine is a science of uncertainty and an art of probability.
—Sir William Osler

Key Points

- Bias is the shorthand way the brain interprets its surroundings.
- Anchoring bias, confirmation bias, diagnostic momentum, and availability heuristic are short-cuts that can distract a physician from considering other causes of a patient's concerns.
- A sensitivity to bias and applying debiasing methods can reduce errors and optimize heuristics.
- The optimal physician-patient interaction recognizes the role of bias in both parties and forges a path to diagnostic accuracy.

Cases

Case 1: History Speaks for Itself

Case 2: The Infection Masquerade

Case 3: Pneumonia in the Time of COVID-19

Cognitive Bias: Inescapable Trap or Integral Tool?

Reality is merely an illusion, albeit a very persistent one.
—Albert Einstein

Human beings peer through lenses of varying degrees of blurriness as they look outside themselves. As much as reality seems genuine, perception influences the experience, making it less concrete. Can we ever share the same understanding of reality if each person views something from an innately distinct perspective?

Rooted in perception is **cognitive bias**. The term applies to subconscious, flawed decision-making that affects how someone comprehends an event, fact, or another person (Cambridge Dictionary). You can think of bias as the brain's adaptation for predicting current circumstances by drawing inferences based on memories. Essentially, our past colors how we live our present; **we see what we expect.**

How does bias affect a doctor-patient visit? Even from the beginning, everyone subconsciously scans appearance, dress, skin color, profession, and communication style—both sender and receiver filter objective observations through a subjective lens.

For physicians, bias impacts interpreting each word and drawing conclusions with incomplete experience and data.

Studies evaluating bias using the Inventory of Cognitive Biases in Medicine (ICBM) suggest that it frequently occurs in clinical practice. With a lower score indicating more bias, pre-clinical medical students scored the lowest (41%) and practicing physicians did only slightly better (49%) (Hershberger, 1996). Ironically, tests that attempt to quantify bias, such as the ICBM, are prone to bias and problems with validity (Sladek, 2008).

Nevertheless, bias does not relegate us to a state of helplessness. We can fortify our interpretative skills and fine-tune our brains to look for patterns through mental shortcuts or heuristics. Furthermore, doctor-doctor and doctor-patient collaborations enhance comprehension and mitigate bias, allowing a greater chance to uncover the cause of a patient's concerns. This chapter will discuss 1) the factors contributing to diagnostic accuracy, 2) the most common types of bias, and 3) ways medical students and physicians can harness the brain's modes of thinking to improve diagnostic yield.

Listen to the Patient

Sir William Osler, considered by many the father of modern medicine, stated, "Listen to your patient. He is telling you the diagnosis." Studies on medical history-taking support this claim. A physician can arrive at a diagnosis from a thorough history around 70 to 90% of the time (Hampton, 1975). Unfortunately, listening to a patient's report does not always yield a clear, undisputed solution. The detection requires a clinician's acumen— a combination of knowledge, experience, dynamic listening, and healthy doses of curiosity and self-doubt.

An interview, or patient history, remains the gateway to an accurate medical diagnosis and treatment. Medical school is a time for the pupil to build and hone these skills. To a physician, an interview is like a trusted tool. Indeed, physicians develop proficiency in this practice. In the span of their careers, they conduct around 100,000 to 200,000 patient interviews (Nichols, 1998).

A clinic visit is not as predictable as a car inspection. The exchange between patient and doctor often encounters roadblocks to interpretation. Vague memories fragment any semblance of an accurate recall. How a patient interacts with their condition may alter the story. The way a physician interprets these words will affect the conclusions. Somewhere within these interactions lies the truth, though both patient and physician change it every step of the way: the disease perception, recollection, communication, assessment, and management.

Physicians carry an added burden since their decisions can impact one's life. A patient seeks consultation with a doctor for assistance and to better understand the "why?" and the "what next?" They may have an idea and would like confirmation. They may suspect a cause that does not fit entirely with online help. They may have researched their symptoms, and cancer remained among hundreds of other plausible reasons.

And why, in this era of internet searches and "Dr. Google," do we still need doctors? When studies evaluated symptom checkers for their accuracy using standardized patients, a correct diagnosis was listed first in 34% of evaluations and in the top 20 diagnoses 58% of the time (Semigran, 2015). Not bad, you may think. Physicians listed the correct diagnosis first (72% vs. 34%) or in the top three (84.3% vs. 51.2%) more often than symptom checkers (Semigran, 2016). On the other hand, they made an incorrect diagnosis in 15% of the cases.

Computer algorithms might help provide options and improve accuracy, but they are not enough. The foundation of clinical diagnosis requires a connection between a patient and a doctor, who envisions the patient's perspective through active listening and clarification. Equally important is that a doctor cannot diagnose a problem simply by troubleshooting detached complaints. To optimize accuracy, they must synthesize concerns and garner individual risk factors and observations. In so doing, skills in pattern detection become the tools.

The availability of medical information allows individuals to be active participants in their care. Access to health websites can be the first step to gaining insight into a medical condition and determining whether a formal visit is required. Likely, information will lead to improved doctor-patient relationships, as patients become more informed and can better describe their conditions and negotiate their care plans (Swee-Lin Tan, 2017).

Case 1: History Speaks for Itself

An ER physician evaluated a 60-year-old man for lower abdominal quadrant pain. He became concerned enough to order a computed tomography (CT) study and bloodwork. The white blood cell count was slightly high at 11 (normal is 4 to 10). Could this be from an early infection?

The scan revealed a sigmoid colon with many diverticula, tiny pockets in the membrane of the colon, and mild, nonspecific inflammation. The radiologist dictated that "there is a possible early diverticulitis," an infection of this tissue. In response to this report, the patient received an antibiotic prescription after being deemed safe for discharge.

I saw the patient in clinic the day after the ER visit. I tuned into the patient's story, asked follow-up questions, and reviewed chart notes. Prior documentation can provide a glimpse into how a physician perceives a patient's history. The notes can shed light on a doctor's inputs and conclusions. In this case, it seemed like the physician was concerned about a more serious condition.

The symptoms were specific to his body position, especially after getting up. Next, I performed a physical examination to confirm the location of the pain and was surprised that the pain was not in the abdomen as the notes indicated; instead, it was in the right groin. I reviewed the CT scan with another radiologist who mentioned it was a "soft call[4]." Sometimes diverticulosis can cause mild inflammation without acute diverticulitis. Antibiotics are not necessary in these cases (Cerosoli, 2018). My impression was that the CT scan was most likely true, and the pain was true, but they were unrelated.

In contrast to the ER diagnosis, I heard a different story. I determined that the pain was in the groin and worsened after abdominal muscle contraction. He had a muscle pull. After I gave my opinion and asked him if he had any questions or comments, the patient remembered that he was building a retaining wall the day before the onset of the pain. He forgot to mention it in the ER. There was enough reason to stop the antibiotics and monitor his steady improvement. Even though physicians have tools to work up problems, sometimes it just takes a listening and curious ear to zero in on the cause.

Case 2: The Infection Masquerade

A fifty-year-old female with obesity saw her primary physician for leg swelling. She woke up and noticed her right lower leg was red and swollen. She recalled bumping it against the bed frame while getting up to use the bathroom at night. She did not experience any fever or chills. The doctor examined her and sent her to the ER out of concern for the leg's appearance.

After the ER evaluation, the team admitted her to the hospital for cellulitis. This condition develops after bacteria invade the skin. Cellulitis can present as a severe infection with sepsis. Her leg was swollen, red, and painful, but she did not have a fever or systemic symptoms. The doctors prescribed her intravenous (IV) antibiotics in the hospital out of concern. Her leg color and size gradually improved. The hospital team discharged her with oral antibiotics for one week. In the clinic follow-up, she stated that the redness came back. The doctor readmitted her to the hospital. She received a few days of IV antibiotics; a nurse placed a central line for ongoing therapy.

The primary care doctor referred her to an infectious disease specialist (me), a physician with two additional years of clinical training in infection management. I listened to the patient as she described the events that led to her visit. I held any comments to avoid interruption and to support her flow. She did not recall ever having any red streaks up her leg, a fever, or shaking chills. Yes, she had ongoing pain from the swelling. No, she had never tried compression stockings.

I considered her presentation from its beginning and thought about cause and effect. Could her improvement on antibiotics in the hospital have been a coincidence? Would other measures alone have improved the redness and swelling? Could this be a situation where bias might have misled physicians to use long-term IV antibiotics?

I reflected on her exam findings in my office: she had swelling in not one but both legs with varying degrees of redness and warmth. Patients who are overweight or have obesity can develop more significant redness and swelling in their legs following trauma. It can be painful and masquerade as cellulitis. Having seen various presentations of this condition, I considered an alternative diagnosis.

I clarified her history that the swelling and redness coincided with an injury.

Upon confirming my suspicions, I took a deep breath as I began to form words that would contradict the conclusions of multiple doctors who saw her previously. I informed her that she did not have an infection. Although she initially expressed concern about the discrepancy, she felt secure with the connection and relieved by the recommendations. She informed me that she felt heard and understood— an essential step in developing rapport and addressing patient fears. I dressed her legs with compression wraps and took her IV line out before she left the clinic. She continued with the dressings to manage the leg swelling and it resolved.

Case 3: Infection in the Time of COVID-19

A family brought a 42-year-old female to the emergency department for worsening shortness of breath and fatigue— both developing over several weeks. The hospitalist contacted me to see the patient and determine if there was anything else to consider. I examined the patient, who was intubated and unable to converse. I reviewed her chart, lab results, and the CT images. The images of her lungs showed "ground-glass[5]" changes, a finding that could be seen with COVID-19.

It appeared we were missing something in the work-up thus far. Two bronchial samples for COVID-19 PCR[6] were negative. The duration did not match the typical period of developing severe COVID-19. Her liver disease meant that she was immunocompromised. All this would make a perfect storm for an opportunistic infection or tuberculosis (TB) reactivation. I recommended that bronchial samples be sent for TB along with other organisms. Both the TB PCR and smear came back positive for tuberculosis. Fortunately, she was a COVID Person Under Investigation (PUI) and was kept in isolation and airborne precautions. These measures protected the hospital staff from tuberculosis exposure from the time she entered the hospital. She was promptly started on TB therapy.

Bias and Its Effect on Medical Practice

Seasoned physicians might be aware of the influence of bias, but no one is immune from it. Medical decisions must transcend the limitations of their perspectives. How do physicians decide accurately? Psychologists Stanovich and West proposed two ways of making decisions: system 1 relates to rapid, intuitive decisions, and system 2 involves slower, more analytical determinations (Stanovich, 2000; Kahneman, 2011). System 2 assesses things more accurately but takes a significant cognitive effort. Conversely, the brain favors system 1 because it is fast yet predictive. Psychologists believe that most people spend about 95% of their time in system 1 thinking (Lakoff, 1999).

You should consider each system as neither good nor bad. Both modes offer advantages in cognition, but either can be associated with distortion and inaccuracy. All decision-making, including in medicine, comes with the risk of cognitive bias, over 32 types (Croskerry, 2003). And more than one can occur at the same time. I will cover the four most common types of bias in medicine.

Common types of bias in medicine

1) Anchoring bias
2) Confirmation bias
3) Diagnosis momentum
4) Availability heuristic

Anchoring bias refers to settling on a diagnosis early on and considering it in future decisions, including treatment (Rounds, 2016). It occurs when a person relies too heavily on the initial information to make decisions. They may discard the history and exam elements that do not fit their original conclusions and order tests to err on the side of caution. A similar type of bias occurs when someone's practice style focuses on the worst-case scenarios, an **attentional bias**. Doctors may anchor their diagnosis too firmly on the "what if," known as a rule-out-the-worst-case-scenario (ROWS) strategy, even though tests contradict it (Croskerry, 2002).

In **Case 1**, the ER doctor began the workup for diverticulitis because of abdominal pain, even though the patient had right groin pain. Another typical example is when a doctor manages a patient with shortness of breath. They may consider a CT angiogram that requires contrast to evaluate for a pulmonary embolism (PE.) A PE is a potentially life-threatening blood clot in the lungs, and it does not always follow a "classic picture." Fortunately, blood tests, heuristic tools, and point-of-care ultrasounds increase diagnostic accuracy and reduce overtesting (e.g., PERC Rule, YEARS algorithm, negative D-dimer) (Bhamidipati, 2021).

Confirmation bias occurs when a physician looks for symptoms or findings characteristic of a particular diagnosis and confirms their original suspicion, rather than weighing in on factors that discredit it. This bias also occurs when any improvement is attributed to the treatment. In **Case 2**, although the patient's leg redness improved after receiving an antibiotic, other treatments, including leg dressings and bedrest, may have been responsible. Confirmation bias likely played a role in **Case 3**, when a doctor may have used the CT findings to support their initial concern about COVID-19.

Diagnosis momentum is a frequent type of cognitive distortion that occurs in medicine. In this bias, doctors fit a patient's presentation in a rubric after the initial assessment without revisiting it (Elston, 2019). Others may continue with the initial diagnosis, not clarifying the history themselves with the patient. The patient with "cellulitis" told the initial physician that she had hit her leg the night before. She also had never had a fever, which frequently accompanies cellulitis. She may have had reduced leg swelling and redness simply by remaining in her bed during the hospitalization. While at home, the swelling and redness may have worsened because she spent more time on her feet. Similarly, **premature closure** relates to finalizing a diagnosis with limited data. This tendency leads to "when the diagnosis is made, the thinking stops" (Croskerry, 2003).

The **availability heuristic** is a form of bias where a more significant probability is applied to one condition just because it quickly comes to mind. Medical schools and residency training will familiarize doctors with common presentations of common illnesses. Physicians learn early on to think of "common things being common," or "when you hear the hoofbeats, think of horses, not zebras," when asked to consider the range of possibilities in the differential diagnosis (Helwig, 1964). It intends to offset the availability heuristic by reminding us to factor in probability more than availability, e.g., what we think about first (Stiegler, 2014).

However, probability alone does not guarantee a diagnosis. In the past few years, radiologists have become adept at interpreting characteristic CT scan patterns in patients with COVID-19 pneumonia, which is the subject of several studies (Shi et al., 2020; Wang et al., 2020). In **Case 3**, the radiologist applied a greater weight in considering COVID-19 over other conditions like miliary TB or pulmonary lymphoma at the time of a pandemic. Even with a CT's high sensitivity (94%) for this process, it has low specificity[7] (37%) (Kim et al. 2020). A CT scan may pick up COVID-19 infection, but it cannot discern between COVID-19 and other diagnoses. A definitive diagnosis falls outside the limits of radiology.

Patient Bias and Other Forms of Cognitive Distortion

A patient must translate their sensations into comprehensible words. It is sometimes hard to separate objective from subjective. Bias can unknowingly mar the fact-finding task of taking a history. For instance, a patient may come in assuming a diagnosis (anchoring bias), stating, "Doctor, I have had this urinary tract infection (UTI) for more than a month," and not consider other causes for their symptoms. Clarifying questions may be helpful, such as "what do you mean when you say urinary tract infection?"

A person may consider an uncommon diagnosis after reading online about an unusual disease fitting their symptoms even to the point that they may seek treatment based on that narrative—a **confirmation bias**. I occasionally see patients who come for chronic Lyme disease concerns, who have repeatedly negative Western blots— virtually ruling out the diagnosis. In some cases, the office visit time may be insufficient to address the strong bias and consider other possibilities.

It is challenging to remember every vital aspect of history. Hindsight often transforms a memory into something different based on one's concerns or assumption of the possibility, inviting another bias known as **recall bias**. Many people have access to the same medical information that doctors have on the internet. However, the knowledge gained through several minutes or hours of reading does not make a person an expert in a field or dissolve bias. The tendency to overrate newly acquired knowledge is the **Dunning-Kruger Effect**. We have seen this effect surface in anti-vaccine sentiment during the pandemic and previously faulty associations with vaccines and autism (Motta, 2018; Pullan, 2021).

It is common for people to overestimate their abilities—**overconfidence bias** while not believing they are. We hear of studies where participants rank their knowledge or skills on driving or good jokes. Most people rank themselves above average, which is statistically impossible (Kruger, 1999). And if you are not convinced that you have bias, you may be under the spell of the **blind spot bias**, when people think they are not prone to as many biases as others (West, 2012). Humans tend not to know what they do not know, and even though the gap closes with knowledge and experience, we cannot escape bias— nor do we need to. The trick is to embrace it.

Methods to Reduce Cognitive Bias

How can doctors and patients avoid these bias traps? First, it is helpful to remember that bias is a natural way the brain manages an inordinate amount of data. Croskerry refers to bias as *Cognitive Dispositions to Respond* (CDR) to emphasize that all cognition uses predictable short-cuts, such as the types described in this chapter. Healthcare would benefit from removing the stigma of bias and developing strategies to optimize decision-making and reduce errors (Croskerry, 2013).

Cognitive debiasing strategies can be excellent starting points to temper the influence of bias. They begin with education and awareness of frequent forms of clinical decision-making bias. Programs can instruct students and residents on cognitive forcing strategies to switch from system 1 to system 2 mode. Slowing down the decision process ("stop, think, then act"), mental checklists, and considering a broader differential diagnosis are some ways to do this (Ely, 2011).

A self-assessment process known as **metacognition**, or "thinking about thinking," underlies these debiasing strategies. It provides a behavioral framework for becoming aware of the influence of bias (Colbert et al., 2015). Metacognitive awareness requires two components: 1) knowledge of cognition and 2) awareness of cognition. Beginning with self-reflection on the thought process, a person determines if it is system 1 or system 2 thinking. Next, they consider the impact of cognitive distortion on the conclusions. The person then enacts debiasing strategies to reapproach these thoughts.

In the medical setting, when metacognition incorporates group collaboration and feedback, it can often guide the team to making better decisions. Ultimately, it teaches individuals to make lasting changes in their behaviors. As an added benefit, practicing metacognition affords a physician empathic listening skills as they consider alternative angles. Medical schools can proactively incorporate these skills early in their curricula[8].

Heuristics and Clinical Decision-Making

The cases in this chapter illustrate the impact of bias on attempts to make objective decisions. Nurses who triage patients with abdominal pain (**Case 1**), leg swelling (**Case 2**), or shortness of breath (**Case 3**) must select from limited data to come up with a potential diagnosis. Next, the physician dives into the history and examination more deeply, applying short-cut rules and knowledge. They weigh possibilities and decide on a diagnosis and treatment plan. All the while, they must acknowledge patients who have concerns about being heard, understood, and feeling better.

When a patient presents[9] with shortness of breath, the physician begins a process of evaluating for causes, such as pulmonary embolism, acute congestive heart failure, acute renal failure, pneumonia, or a panic attack. Some of these are potentially life-threatening, while others are not. A clinician then ranks the most likely diagnoses based on the elements of the history, physical examination, and other studies and works toward a plan, including further tests and treatments, e.g., ordering a chest radiograph or ordering a 2-D echo to evaluate the heart valves. After these tests return, physicians sift through the barrage of data to see if the results satisfy the working diagnosis. If not, they must reframe their understanding and consider other possibilities. Thus, medical decision-making is a dynamic interplay involving the patient, the physician, and data.

However, we decide in a context of bias and behavior. A doctor's past training or experience, missing a diagnosis, "being burned," or having a malpractice claim may affect the attention attached to specific complaints or findings. The rationale of "just in case" or "CYA[10]" can expose patients to unnecessary testing and treatment and increase costs and risks.

Even ordering an extra test can affect medical decision-making and prompt further needless testing. Medication prescribing falls in this bucket. Programs like antibiotic stewardship aim to foster judicious prescribing with evidence and collaborative decision-making to reduce antibiotic overuse, side effects, and resistance. Their strategies benefit from a solid understanding of bias (Langford, 2020).

How do we navigate to a decision amid uncertainty? Cognition fills in the gaps by considering what cannot be determined until there is an acceptable solution. Herbert Simon, regarded as the father of artificial intelligence, described the concept of bounded rationality in the context of decision-making. He proposed that humans rationalize a good enough or satisficing solution from "sufficing" and "satisfying," factoring in what is known and unknown. These efforts aim to simplify the process while not compromising accuracy. The brain does this through heuristics, or cognitive shortcuts—system 1 decisions. It is a way to reduce what would otherwise be unmanageable data (Marewski, 2012).

Heuristics are formalized mental pathways that approach a clinical dilemma with a best-fit estimate (Marewski, 2012). These evidence-based systems simplify decision-making and are used frequently in the form of tools and checklists in healthcare. One example is a dosing nomogram that pharmacists can follow to adjust medications and reduce the risk of harm. Other tools are *fast-and-frugal-heuristics*, which often employ binary (yes or no) decision pathways to reach a diagnosis or triage plan with less information (Marewski, 2012). *Fast-and-frugal* trees include heart attack triage starting with ECG changes (**Figure 2** above), syphilis screening using Treponemal antibodies, and when to perform a CT to rule out a lung blood clot.

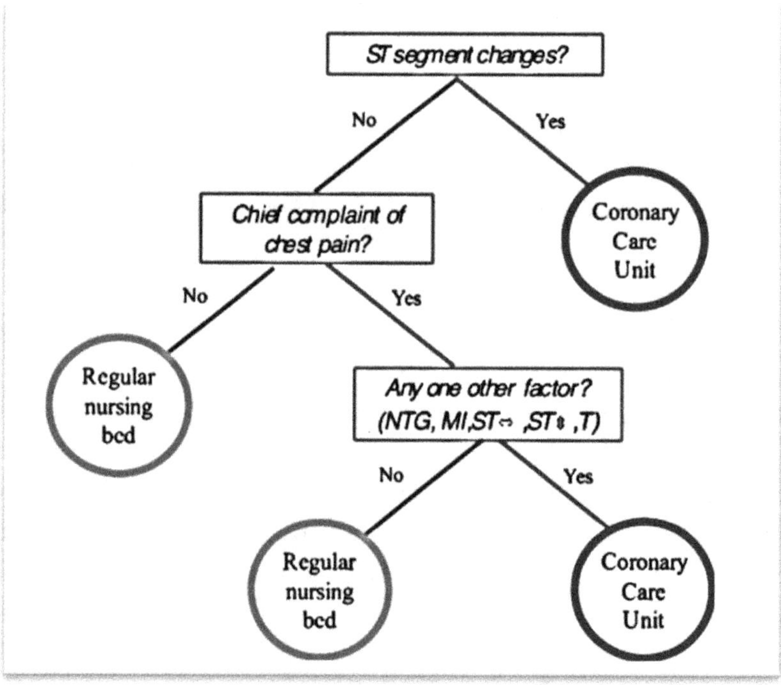

Figure 2: A fast-and-frugal tree for ER doctors to decide where to admit a patient (Green & Mehr, 1997)

Knowledge Gaps, Bias, and Diagnostic Considerations

The mind more commonly goes to system 1 thinking, relying on intuition, experience, and pattern-finding. It is a beneficial skill that can be honed but often overlooks its blind spots and invites bias. The rubric of common things occur commonly reminds students to stay grounded in their differential diagnosis[11]. But rubrics can neither fill in holes nor capture exceptions.

As a student, I thought, as many do, that devoting more time to knowledge building was going to shield me from making mistakes and potentially harming patients. I struggled with how I would manage knowledge gaps as I became a physician. Unlike one textbook for each college course, multiple references, articles, study aids, and online resources can be overwhelming for medical students. I convinced myself that sitting and studying 6 to 8 hours a day would seal those gaps.

I combined my two fascinations through medical school and residency: learning and travel. I wondered if working in developing countries could give me a context to "fill in the missing pieces" of my knowledge, like a chapter on tropical medicine or a rare disease that no one ever remembers. However, these experiences allowed me to reflect on my thinking and practice making decisions in diverse settings rather than fill the knowledge bucket.

Back to the *think horses, not zebras* principle: my usual disclaimer is except when you are in Africa. When you hear hoofs, consider zebras, but do not forget to consider an occasional wildebeest or hartebeest. It took a trip to Africa for me to learn to think outside the box. Sometimes what seems like the most probable cause is an unlikely one masquerading. A diagnosis is not a probability but an actuality.

When formulating a differential diagnosis list, certain factors in the history guide a physician's thoughts. Some pathogens thrive only in specific environments, such as coccidioidomycosis in the Southwestern USA and malaria in the tropics. Other microbes follow exposures, such as thorn pricks (*Sporothrix*) and air conditioner units (*Legionella*). Some diseases occur only in those with risk factors, such as Salmonella osteomyelitis in sickle cell anemia or *Vibrio vulnificus* septicemia in those with cirrhosis.

Physicians-in-training will mostly see common presentations of common diseases and several uncommon presentations of common conditions (**Table 1**). Less frequently, they may even see a common presentation of an uncommon illness, such as malaria or dengue fever. However, physicians will likely encounter an unusual presentation of an uncommon disease during their career — sometimes without realizing it. They may unknowingly try to fit a square peg into a round hole.

Balancing Knowledge Gaps and Heuristics in Medical School

You may wonder how doctors learn to make accurate decisions. Does it come from a strong clinical or basic-science background? While a good knowledge base may at first seem crucial for diagnostic accuracy, it does not guarantee that a physician accurately assesses a condition with minimal bias. Knowledge may enhance understanding and the differential diagnosis, but cognitive bias stems from an error in how the brain interprets new information while accessing fragmented memories. Retrospective studies on diagnostic errors show that most occur because of clinical reasoning gaps, such as faulty synthesis or premature closure, rather than fund of knowledge issues (Graber, 2005).

Not to mention that medical schools find it increasingly challenging to keep up with the literature. As students race to review the latest information, researchers publish new articles. Present estimates for doubling time of medical knowledge seem

Table 1: Range of Clinical Presentations

Common presentation/ common illness	Uncommon presentation/ common illness
Influenza with flu symptoms	Influenza myocarditis
Pneumococcal Lobar pneumonia	Pneumonia with empyema
DVT with pulmonary embolism	DVT with paradoxical stroke from patent foramen
Chlamydia cervicitis	Chlamydia with Fitz-Hugh-Curtis syndrome
Common presentation/ uncommon illness	**Uncommon presentation/ uncommon illness**
Ascending Guillain-Barre Syndrome	Miller-Fisher variant of Guillain-Barre Syndrome
Malaria with fever and hemolysis	Cerebral Malaria
Classic Dengue Fever	Dengue Hemorrhagic Fever

insurmountable. Every few months, the total volume of medical information doubles, when it was every fifty years in the 1950s (Densen, 2011). Knowledge gaps are likely to grow wider as the fund of knowledge expands.

A physician's skill to distinguish a probable explanation from multiple options starts in medical school. Though it may seem knowledge-heavy, students apply heuristics to simplify and make the information relevant. They practice constructing differential diagnoses or rank order lists of plausible causes. They develop methods to discern worst-case scenarios from less likely ones.

There are mnemonics for the cranial nerves, checklists for risk factors in conditions like post-operative infections, blood clots, and gallbladder disease, and flashcards that review a disease's key points.

Medical students and residents have structured clinical time to gain operational experience, feedback, and decision-making skills. The future doctor has an opportunity to develop behaviors that employ system 1 and system 2 decisions beneficially. Training alongside supervising physicians, residents, and peers affords a greater group[12] awareness of the process of deciding. For accurately ranking the top diagnoses, one study found that even groups as small as two doctors benefited compared to individual physicians. The researchers referred to this as collective intelligence (Barnett, 2019).

Consequently, some psychologists recommend that medical schools develop decision-making curricula featuring group learning, feedback, and instruction to maximize heuristics rather than avoiding the "elephant in the room." Schools should prioritize collaborative exploration, evidence-based practices, short-hand rules, and feedback to train students to make better decisions and "smarter" mistakes (Feufel, 2019).

Summary

The brain performs a best-fit attempt to fill in the gaps between what is known and what is not. The brain acts as a code breaker, but the same skillset that decodes can also obfuscate. Correctly diagnosing a disease entails turning down "the white noise" of bias.

In the clinic, the patient and physician take turns listening and speaking. The inner experience of the unfolding symptoms of a patient gets translated into selected spoken words. Each word carries a message yet has limitations. Both individuals attempt to find meaning in words. Bias can enter every step of the exchange.

Methods that strengthen collective decision-making and increase awareness, such as metacognition, can improve care and reduce medical errors.

A distressing feature in the life which you are about to enter, a feature which will press hardly upon the finer spirits among you and ruffle their equanimity, is the uncertainty which pertains not alone to our science and art, but to the very hopes and fears which make us (humans). In seeking absolute truth, we aim at the unattainable and must be content with finding broken portions.

—Sir William Osler

CHAPTER 4

On Medical Errors

Progress through trial and error depends not only on making trials but also on recognizing errors.
-Virginia Postrel

Key Points

- Medical errors often result from bias.
- Errors can be reduced through patient collaboration, considering a differential diagnosis, and self-care.

Cases

- Case 4: It was in the Decimal Point (Prescribing Error)
- Case 5: Postoperative Foot Pain (False Attribution)
- Case 6: Postoperative Increased White Blood Cell Count (Surgical Miscount Error)
- Case 7: Treating to Cover the Bases (Mistaken Diagnosis and Specialist Bottleneck)

Introduction: Errors are a Significant Health Risk

Students pay particular attention to literature for examinations and bolster their knowledge base during medical school. However, they must accept that there will still be cognitive bias no matter how intensive the didactic training is. And making a mistake as a doctor has more significant consequences than getting a wrong answer on a test.

The impact of errors in healthcare is under-appreciated—statistics on death certificates only factor in disease conditions and not medical errors. When taken into account, they are the *third leading cause of death in the US*, with an estimated quarter-million people dying each year[13] (Markary, 2016). The source in the majority (78.9%) were cognitive errors; a lower percentage (13%) was from the misinterpretation of results (Singh, 2013). This information is not intended to frighten readers. It is a reminder that errors occur in medical practice, and most physicians will make many small ones and a few large ones during their careers. Although mistakes in medicine are common, the likelihood of severe errors is low.

As discussed in Chapter 3, we all make errors in cognition. Experience is often the best teacher. A physician learns to make decisions, navigate successfully toward the diagnosis, re-evaluate conclusions, and recalibrate if needed. Nevertheless, errors will happen. It is also helpful to view them as shared learning opportunities, although the medical field does not always embrace the benefits of this dialogue.

Several things can decrease the risk and impact of medical errors. This chapter aims to inform the reader how to approach healthcare mindfully and become more aware and proactive. Firstly, I would like to share some of the experiences that made an impression on me and that I still remember all too vividly.

Case 4: It was in the Decimal Point

The intern year marks the transition from an observer role to an active participant in a patient's care. Interns carry responsibilities such as the data gatherer, order writer, care communicator, patient advocate, discharge organizer, and the first doctor to see and evaluate a patient. Interns begin the day by visiting patients before rounding with their residents and attendings. They review vital signs, meds from the medication administration records (MAR), and lab and culture results from computer databases. The time gives them a chance to troubleshoot and construct a plan before communicating with the team. A team consists of several medical students, two to three interns, a second-year resident (R2), a senior resident (R3), and the attending physician overseeing them.

Interns and residents typically have one continuity clinic weekly, leaving the team to cover each other's patients. There is not always a guarantee that someone covering can accomplish the same tasks as the assigned intern. The details could get omitted from intern to resident to attending as more senior members often focus on evaluation and treatment strategies rather than an intern's tasks. *But the devil is in the details*—in this case, the MAR chart. An ideal setting would be to check it every day, ensuring correct dosages. Also, in the nineties, hospital pharmacy departments did not have the same checks and balances as in this era of electronic records and more extensive PharmD management.

On rounds, I received a new patient. She was an elderly woman admitted overnight for "adult failure to thrive[14]," and screening tests showed hypothyroidism, enough that we decided to start her on therapy. Levothyroxine (T4) is a synthetic thyroid hormone that is a metabolic stimulant and keeps the body functioning normally in those with thyroid problems.

The usual way to start someone on therapy is to initiate 25 micrograms a day and increase gradually over several weeks until reaching an effective dose, usually between 75 to 150 micrograms. The thyroid-stimulating hormone (TSH) level, released by the anterior pituitary gland when there is a metabolic need for more T4, can be checked periodically, usually after weeks of replacement therapy.

Most medications are milligrams in size (1 x 10^{-3}grams). The body only needs microgram doses (1 x 10^{-6} grams) of thyroid replacement. After reciting that I would give 25 micrograms, I wrote the wrong dose— using one less zero before the number. The quantity I wrote was 0.25 mg instead of 0.025 milligrams, an amount of 250 micrograms instead of 25 micrograms.

225 micrograms (225 x 10^{-6} grams) may seem like an insignificant amount, but it is a tenfold difference. Before writing the order, I translated the dose of 25 micrograms into milligrams and forgot the correct format. In today's setting of electronic orders, an error such as this would not be likely. It would have flagged the pharmacist, if not the prescriber, first.

The next day was my short day, and my R2 covered for me. He did not catch the mistake. I returned the day after but ran out of time before rounds to review the MAR. By the time we found the dosage error, she had already received six doses of the 250 micrograms.

When I discovered it, I felt that feeling in the pit of my stomach as the shame surfaced. I searched for explanations: maybe I should have rechecked it on my "peripheral brain" (the pharmacopeia booklet in my white coat); my R2 covering for me should have reviewed the MAR while preparing the note. However, there was no escaping that I was responsible for this error.

We transferred her to the telemetry ward for heart rate monitoring. And, yes, she had an **adverse event** after getting too high of a dose. She developed tachycardia[15] and brief runs of atrial fibrillation. It prolonged her hospitalization for another week. I processed how my error affected someone's health and appreciated how forgiving my colleagues and supervisors were - and the patient herself. I realized that an error does not define someone. I let go of its hold on me as I slowly eased into a post-error me. I made a habit of reviewing the order plans before and after writing them, and I avoided making this kind of error again.

Types of Medical Errors

Cognitive bias leads to the two major types of medical errors: omission and commission. Errors of omissions entail an action not taken to treat or reduce harm, often in the setting of misdiagnosis. As the disease develops, it may lead to further injury or liability, such as not working up a patient with headaches who has early signs of meningitis. An error of commission is mistaken action taken. Occasionally, providers start and continue treatment "just in case," though the diagnosis may still need clarifying. There can also be breakdowns at several points, from the medication order to its administration. If a patient receives an incorrect dose or wrong treatment, it constitutes an error of commission. (Rodziewicz, 2022).

Case 5: Postoperative Foot Pain

Some patients can be challenging, not just because they have cryptic complaints. During my work as a primary care doctor, I treated a man who was a smoker, obese, had diabetes, high blood pressure, and sleep apnea. He also had a history of renal cell carcinoma. Several years after a surgeon removed his left kidney, the oncologist found a small metastatic lung focus on surveillance that required surgical attention. Metastasis means that cancer shows up in a different part of the body. Approximately one-third of patients with renal cell carcinoma have metastatic disease on presentation (Gong, 2016).

He had a complicated past, both medically and in general, but he was also at times very unagreeable and even demanding of the staff. He told me that he trusted almost no one and kept a gun in his house in case he decided "to end it." After getting to know him, I realized that it was as much a part of his dark humor as it was probably true. He confided in me about his concerns, fears, and even his sordid past. He had a way of going through all his troubles that made his visits last longer than most patients. I gave him the time but often found myself running behind schedule on his appointment days.

He was approved for bariatric surgery after he successfully quit smoking. He wanted to lose weight, alleviate his medical conditions, and find love. After many years of being unhealthy, he told me he was "sick of being sick." A few days after the surgery, I visited him in the hospital, and he informed me things went well. I called him a few weeks later, and he mentioned some of his fears about his health and mood after surgery.

I saw him in the office the following month. Among several concerns was a pain in his left foot near the ankle, which he mentioned at the visit's end. I speculated that it might be from overuse since he was walking more. I recommended we address it at a follow-up visit if it continued.

A month later, his foot was still hurting, and it was not only associated with walking. I gave him some ankle exercises but told him it might require more tests. Four months passed. After coming in for bloodwork, he was still in pain and needed a visit. The nurse informed me of his status, and we ordered foot X-rays in advance.

We focused on the ongoing pain when he came in the next time. I noted that he had lost substantial weight and looked healthier. We discussed the results of the foot films. They showed an unexpected finding: a lytic lesion (near-broken bone) of his fibula. A development such as this was a red flag of an essential part of his health history that I had overlooked when he mentioned foot pain: his renal cell carcinoma.

Many thoughts rushed through my mind. I felt vulnerable and exposed because I had missed the early clues over two visits. I falsely attributed the pain to a muscular or tendinous process, and, in this setting, X-rays are not usually beneficial. Admittedly, my initial reaction was to search elsewhere for responsibility. Could the oncology group have forgotten to address the musculoskeletal complaints in the follow-up visits, even after the surveillance CT scans of his thorax, abdomen, and pelvis were negative? Should he have come in more frequently, so we could have just spoken about the foot? Whatever the case, I found myself in the crosshairs of an *error of omission.*

I promptly called an oncologic orthopedic surgeon at the referral hospital and got him scheduled for a visit. They ordered a bone biopsy with radiology, and the pathology of the sample confirmed renal cell carcinoma. A few weeks later, he had surgery and had the distal fibula resected.

He came back to my office with his girlfriend for a follow-up visit. He required a cane for support. I apologized to him for the delay in the diagnosis, and he accepted my apology and acknowledgment. On a later visit, he mentioned that his girlfriend told him to sue me. He reflected on it and disagreed since he appreciated our solid doctor-patient relationship. We discussed the missed opportunities, including not taking enough time in earlier visits to address the pain and the long gaps between visits.

Clear objectives need to be set at the beginning of the visit to ensure that each issue is addressed with enough time and detail to decide the next steps. Additionally, even though someone has a specialist, e.g. an oncologist, patients are more likely to report a new concern to their primary care doctor. It was surprising that the diagnosis only needed an X-ray to confirm it. I will never forget the importance of open dialogue, close follow-up, and a focused history and examination.

Missed Cancer Diagnosis

Almost half of diagnostic errors (46%) in the primary care setting occur from a missed diagnosis of cancer. The most frequently overlooked include lung, colorectal, prostate, and breast. Clinical decisions, such as delaying or not ordering a test made up most errors (51%), while a referral delay was second (37%) (Aaronson, 2019). As cancer is best treated when it is identified earlier, a missed or delayed diagnosis often has significant repercussions. In the setting of the pandemic, there was a disruption in routine cancer screening, with reductions up to 90% for colon and 85% for breast, which could have dire ramifications for patients (Patt, 2020).

Case 6: Postoperative Increased White Blood Cell Count

One of the more common consults for an infectious disease service is to evaluate someone with an increased white blood cell (WBC) count. A WBC count is primarily elevated from inflammation, whether the cause is infectious or non-infectious.

The patient was a woman who needed emergency abdominal surgery for a perforated cholecystitis, i.e., a ruptured gallbladder. Postoperatively, she developed a fever and a doubling of her white count from 12,000 (normal is >4,000 and <10,000) to 24,000. The surgeon did not report any obvious intraoperative complications other than minimal leakage of infected gallbladder contents. The patient was kept on antibiotics until they could clarify the source of the count.

Surgeons often ask an infectious disease doctor to see a post-surgical patient for fever and a high WBC count. The mnemonic, "the five W's," capture some of the causes. These are "wind" for pneumonia, "walk" for blood clots in the leg, "wound" for wound infection, "water" for urinary tract infection, and "wonder drug" for medication fever.

The examination did not suggest another site or cause other than the abdomen. It is not unusual to have a fever and white blood cell count after abdominal surgery, but this was concerning. If the count worsens after surgery, prompt re-imaging of the abdomen with a CT scan may be necessary.

The next day, her WBCs increased to 36,000, and she had a persistent fever. I ordered a CT scan. There were some post-op changes in the right upper quadrant of the abdomen, so the radiologist had difficulty interpreting the findings in that area. Another day later, the WBC increased to 40,000. It was time to decide whether the abdomen needed to be explored. The surgeon took her back to the OR and discovered a retained surgical gauze in the patient's abdomen. After removing the gauze, the patient's blood count levels and temperatures normalized.

Retained Surgical Bodies

Retained surgical bodies (RSB) include surgical instruments, needles, electrodes, and gauzes and occur at an estimated rate of 0.3 to 1.0 per 1,000 abdominal surgeries. If we factor in more than 28 million operations in the US yearly, this represents about 1,500 cases. Of all types of RSB, the most common are sponges left at the surgical site. Risk factors for this misadventure include the complexity of the surgery, obesity, and trauma. Interestingly, the team confirmed a "correct" surgical sponge count in 80 percent of the retained sponge cases (Zejnullahu, 2017).

Case 7: Treating to Cover the Bases

Some time ago, I saw a patient in the hospital for an infectious disease consultation with multiple nonspecific complaints, including loss of coordination and trouble walking. He reported seizure-like activity. He had no prior history of medical conditions or obvious risk factors.

There was enough concern to prompt a brain CT scan and MRI. The CT scan suggested a developing process with multiple findings made more apparent on the follow-up MRI. These were **demyelinating** lesions: spots in the brain tissue where neurons are inflamed and damaged. There were numerous small lesions, some of them ring-enhancing. This appearance sometimes suggests infections.

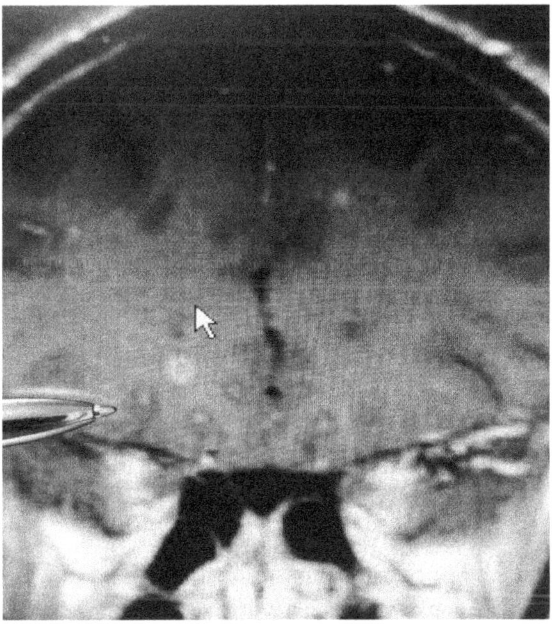

Figure 1. Coronal View of the Patient's MRI Demonstrating Multiple Lesions

The radiologist provided a differential diagnosis, including multiple sclerosis (MS) and a parasitic infection known as neurocysticercosis[16] (NC). Neurocysticercosis is a condition caused by larvae that migrate to the brain after the ingestion of foods contaminated with the cysts of the tapeworm *Taenia solium* (Mewara, 2013). A neurologist saw the patient and was surprised by the extent of the lesions for MS. He speculated about alternative diagnoses.

Was this my first case of neurocysticercosis in the United States? Conferring directly with the neurologist and radiologist offered no further clarification. An additional review from the MRI did not provide any additional information than what it already suggested (**Figure 1**). Although I had doubts about any parasitic infection, I ordered blood NC antibodies, expecting them to be negative[17], and recommended considering a lumbar puncture to rule out MS[18]. The patient declined the procedure because he was concerned about things he had to do and left against medical advice (AMA).

One week later, I saw him in the clinic. He had no obvious risk factor for NC. Adding confusion to the case was that the NC serologic test returned positive. I needed more information to make a diagnosis, but arranging a lumbar puncture and neurologist follow-up was challenging. I contacted the neurologist's partner with whom I often collaborated. He told me that his schedule was overbooked, and he could not fit him in for several weeks.

With the positive test, I wondered what harm would occur if I treated him with a few doses of albendazole, an anti-parasitic agent, and prednisone while awaiting the additional tests and procedure. Prednisone is used in NC to reduce inflammation while on the treatment. I realized that this might be beneficial if it were MS, but it was not a long-term option. He could not walk well and used a walker. I sympathized with his situation.

I reminded the patient that we did not make a definitive diagnosis and referred him for a lumbar puncture. With his situation and the delays, I convinced myself to treat him while getting him scheduled for a lumbar puncture. Miraculously, two weeks later, he came back much improved on the prednisone and the albendazole.

On his return visit a few weeks later, the earlier improvements dissipated as the prednisone dose decreased, and he was in a comparable situation as before. At this point, there was no other way to do this other than to send him to a referral center for admission. I informed the medical staff of my treatment decisions and recommended additional tests. He was taken to the center the same day with no further delay in his evaluation.

The cerebrospinal fluid was positive for myelin basic protein (MBP). The MRI showed some of the lesions had receded while new ones appeared. These findings strongly suggested the diagnosis of multiple sclerosis. I later read of the association with MS, an autoimmune condition, and false-positive antibody studies, including those for neurocysticercosis.

Diagnostic Error (Misdiagnosis)

Diagnostic error makes up about 14% of all errors and comprises a quarter (26%) of all medicolegal claims (Leape, 1991; CRICO/RMF, 2010). Studies on misdiagnosis categorize errors as "no fault," system-based, and human-cognitive (Neale, 2011). "No fault" errors occur when a disease develops unusually or silently. System errors include technical issues or hospital issues that lead to an error. As discussed previously, cognitive bias has the greatest influence on diagnostic error.

A misdiagnosis can occur for several reasons: attributing an insensitive test as more sensitive than it is (therefore excluding the possibility of a diagnosis in a patient who tested negative); attributing a test to be more specific than it is (and making a diagnosis when it still could be another condition); overemphasizing initial findings and not factoring new results (anchoring bias); working with earlier presumptions without adjusting the differential diagnosis on your exam (errors of commission or omission).

It is advisable to consult openly with specialists. A phone consult can help frame further workups while awaiting a referral visit. Sometimes specialists can get a patient in more quickly after speaking with the primary care physician and getting the bulk of the story.

Patients are responsible for ensuring that they have follow-up visits and begin contacting the specialists. Since a delay in treatment may occur while a patient awaits a visit, it might be tempting for primary care physicians to treat while evaluating. PCPs can weigh options with their patients and err on the side of postponing therapy for more complicated conditions until they are seen by the specialist. If the patient's condition worsens, they may need a hospital admission to accelerate the work-up.

Common Errors in Radiology

It is not the job of the radiologist to diagnose a condition. Radiology does not always provide a definitive diagnosis. It is not uncommon for a radiologist to list a series of possible causes to explain the images. One important consideration is that they often lack thorough historical information and clinical examination findings. If the results are still not specific enough, it should prompt the physician to consider other causes. Some conditions show comparable results on MRI, and clinical correlation is always necessary.

Radiologists are human, too; they can miss or misinterpret findings. Studies suggest that errors are common enough in radiology, with a 3-5% daily error rate (Brady, 2017). Sometimes it is harder to find something else when an order is framed as "rule out X." I will never forget a patient with extreme chest pain and a CT scan of the thorax to evaluate the patient for an aneurysm, a weakened arterial wall at risk for rupture. The radiologist read it as "negative" for a worst-care scenario vascular issue. However, looking for an aneurysm led the radiologist to overlook mediastinal air (that is, within the encasement of the heart) and subtle free air under the diaphragm. The patient had another life-threatening cause, a hole (perforation) in their esophagus.

A radiologist's determinations may be succinct and seem definitive on the report. However, the interpretation may suffer without a clinical context. Clinicians have the most crucial resource for detection: the patient. Clinical information improves radiologists' accuracy and inter-observer consistency (Tudor, 1997). Likewise, a team-based approach to radiology improves care and avoids a missed or mistaken diagnosis.

My immediate reaction was that I had taken a gamble on a patient. Factors included the bottlenecks in all directions, the radiologist's input of "could be neurocysticercosis," and the positive antibody test. On the other hand, I had reached out multiple times to local neurologists and scheduled the admission about six weeks after the initial hospitalization.

He returned to the clinic four weeks after his discharge. He brought in a form for medical marijuana, and, after confirming that MS was an included condition, I promptly approved it. I apologized for the delay and explained to him the challenges. He completely understood and appreciated my assistance in getting him seen.

It can be challenging when patients refuse testing during an evaluation. Sometimes, what is available is still not enough, leaving a doctor searching for a definitive diagnosis. While I enjoy being of service and getting answers for my patients, it is potentially harmful to anchor on a diagnosis with limited information or pending tests. I emerged from the experience with a greater sense of the importance of collaboration in confirming a diagnosis. Occasionally, with more severe conditions, additional tests are needed before treatment. And if there is a bottleneck, sometimes it is reasonable to admit a patient or find another specialist that can see him sooner.

How Doctors Reduce Errors and Move Forward with Greater Certainty

Becoming a physician is an apprenticeship. Medical rotations offer opportunities for students and residents to make decisions that affect patient outcomes while having oversight and feedback from more experienced doctors. The team-based approach provides greater support to reduce errors before writing an order. Meetings can include discussing treatment options, risks, and benefits and can be formal or informal. Nevertheless, some treatments require enough diagnostic certainty because there is an increased potential for harm.

A physician faces uncertainty in diagnosis, and bias can distort a systematic framework. Juxtaposed with this is the momentum of an illness. Harm can follow premature treatment, just as much as leaving conditions to develop until greater urgency arises. Nevertheless, there are ways to prevent or mitigate errors. Some of the most important include 1) communication, 2) trusting but verifying conclusions, 3) staying aware of bias, and 4) self-care.

Communication, Communication, Communication

I cover the importance of communication in **Chapter 8**, but below are a few points related to medical errors. About a quarter of malpractice cases for medical errors (27%) stem from a breakdown in communication (Tiwary, 2019). The claims describe several areas where there was faulty communication. The physician committed an error in thought, whether it was because of something not shared or verified or a step not taken. A patient with abdominal surgery presented with a high WBC in the OR after a surgical sponge miscount. In the patient with MS, there was no clear line of responsibility established – an ID issue versus a neurologist issue.

Collaboration requires open channels of communication. It can be instrumental in determining the diagnosis's momentum and need for treatment, the interpretation of the results, and the need for further work-up. Calling a radiologist or walking down to the reading room can often open a dialogue that enhances patient care and reduces errors. Medications and doses can be discussed, along with follow-up plans. These interactions ensure that the step forward is due diligence and increased coordination.

Diagnosis Benefits from a "Trust but Verify" Mindset

When a covering physician sees a hospitalized patient for the first time, they should review enough history to understand the conclusions but attempt to hold back any diagnosis until they have heard the story directly from the patient. Errors in commission begin with an initial diagnosis carried through into treatment without reconsideration. Remember, the physician's responsibility lies in assisting the patient. The best start and finish come with the patient's account and a proper physical examination. The physician should not leave the rectal examination to the consultant[19].

A physician encounters a diagnosis at the interplay of the patient's presentation and the study results. Medical diagnosis requires sifting through a plethora of information. A physician realizes that test results are sometimes "positive" or "negative," but they must review above the bottom line. For instance, essential information occasionally lies hidden in the descriptions, such as pathology or radiology findings. Other times, the tests may be inaccurate, such as a false positive or false negative. Sometimes a test needs to be repeated at a second timepoint.

Specific lab tests require interpretation and cannot be declared "normal" or "abnormal." For example, I frequently see patients for false-positive HIV tests or positive Lyme disease titers where the provider draws conclusions from the study results[20]. A closer look at the details often shows no such concern. To reduce an error in diagnosis, which can spiral into treatment misadventures, confirm every test result before concluding.

A question to ask: is there enough information to start treatment? As for the medication, is the usual dosage enough, or is it too much for the specific patient to consider liver and kidney function and drug interactions? A doctor takes care to write orders free of distraction and reviews them to ensure they are interpretable, the dosage is correct, and the form of administration is accurate. Newer electronic medical record systems can reduce many order entry errors, including doses, units, drug interactions, drug allergies, and redundancy. A review of reputable online resources or smartphone apps can be beneficial before formulating orders and follow-up plans.

Keep in Mind the Possibility of Bias

A doctor's memory interacts with objective data, allowing them to draw inferences. Even though bias can lead to error, within it is the substance of a seasoned physician. A knowledge base cannot be complete and hermetically sealed. There will always be discoveries, knowledge gaps, and anomalies in real life. Experience may be limited to a few patients with one diagnosis, and these individual presentations may affect how a physician addresses future patients.

Many steps are required to produce a diagnosis. A patient discusses how their body feels and when the dysfunction began. They select words to describe this, which have a subjective value. Is it chest "pain," a feeling of "pressure," or is it "like an elephant sitting on your chest?" Although this could raise concerns about a heart attack, the statements are like raw data that require further processing. What was the context of the pain? Are there any other associated symptoms or findings? Upon closer inspection, the doctor may identify a shingles rash on the patient's chest. Whatever it is, the physician attempts to interpret the words objectively, but subjectivity taints the process.

The physician's skill set requires shaping a framework of possibilities or a differential diagnosis. A degree of skepticism tempers a physician's conclusions, protecting them from anchoring or confirmation bias. The challenge is that a physician may face a rare presentation of a common illness or a rare presentation of a rare illness and only recall from an incomplete experience base.

Bias is an unavoidable result of cogitating. We can only prepare for it and embrace it. Our brains unconsciously relate to current experiences using a past repertoire. Inherent to bias is the risk of miscalculating from limited experience, however ample it may seem. Therefore, particularly with a difficult diagnosis, it is helpful to review the case, either informally with colleagues or formally through consultation.

Self-Care

A common sentiment among physicians, particularly in training, is "work hard, play hard." Although this behavior may sustain one through short-term challenges, it suggests that one extreme nullifies another extreme. Some might construe this as a great reason to drink excess alcohol following a tough work week. What is missing is a message of a balanced lifestyle with plenty of sleep, good nutrition, and exercise to protect oneself from burn-out and fatigue. Burnout and sleep deprivation commonly can lead to cognitive fatigue and a tendency to rely too heavily on heuristics, such as bias (Johnson, 2016). Lack of self-care could impair one's ability to assess a patient objectively and contribute to misdiagnosis and errors.

CHAPTER 5

Generalist and Specialist: Putting the Patient as the Priority

A child looked after by seven nannies is without one eye.
—Russian Proverb

Too many cooks in the pot spoil the broth.
—Anonymous

Key Points

- Primary care physicians play an instrumental role in patient care through health promotion, preventive screening, and chronic disease management.

- There has been a shift toward specialization in the United States, potentially leading to shortages in primary care and increases in healthcare costs.

- A primary care physician serves as a patient's collaborator, advocate, organizer, and expert for health care needs.

- A specialist may focus on one system or approach but benefits by upholding a whole-patient approach.

Cases

Case 8: "Just Need a Refill of My Prescriptions"

Case 9: Multiple Episodes of Pneumonia While on Chemotherapy

Case 10: Having the Heart to Prescribe

Introduction: One Doctor for Each Problem?

Patients navigate through a care model of generalists and specialists within the United States. They are two sides of the same coin, addressing the problems within the same context— a patient's body. Other health problems do not cease when a specialist manages a specific organ system or field. And just because a specialist addresses an issue does not mean that a primary care provider stops thinking about it. The care of the patient is the top priority.

Sometimes it can be difficult to delineate the responsibility of patient care. The aphorisms at the beginning of this chapter can apply to healthcare. As a medical student, I worked with a cardiologist who did primary care. At the time, it was common for specialists to build their practice from the ground up and accept all patients to fill in the gaps. After several years, his cardiology practice was booming, but he continued to see his established patients for general issues.

He referred those patients to other consultants for issues most primary care doctors could address. All his patients with diabetes would go to an endocrinologist. His female patients would go to a gynecologist for routine pap smears. Some patients could have three or more physicians involved in their care. He would treat their cardiology issues, like high blood pressure and atrial fibrillation, but would often focus on these issues over general health concerns during visits. Was seeing several physicians helpful for the patients?

The Growing Shortage of Primary Care Physicians

My experiences in medical school fortified an appreciation of the importance of generalists to patient care. Starting with its location in southern Ohio, my school emphasized primary care in health maintenance and chronic disease management[21]. There are physician shortages in rural areas across all disciplines. Although 20% of the US population lives in a rural setting, only 9% of physicians practice in these areas (Rosenblatt, 2000). Physicians who are highly specialized tend to work at major medical centers in cities. Consequently, it is common in rural settings that primary care doctors often manage the complete health needs of their patients. A strong background in primary care became the foundation of my interest in a comprehensive approach as an internist and infectious diseases specialist.

Is there a shortage of primary care physicians? Compared to 50% in 1961, the percentage of primary care physicians (PCPs) in the United States dropped to 33% in 2015 (AAMC, 2016). That means that two-thirds of physicians-in-training are now seeking a specialization. The Association of American Medical Colleges projects that there will be a shortage of up to 55,200 primary care physicians by the next decade (AAMC, 2020.)

Some of the reasons students choose not to go into primary care include the lower salaries, less practice flexibility in an overburdening electronic health record (EHR), higher levels of burnout, and an increase in medical complexity with less reimbursement. The average overall physician salary was $299,000. Compared with specialists who earned $329,000 annually, primary care physicians, who often have more extended workdays, earned around $223,000 (Medscape, 2018)[22]. Meanwhile, the average medical school debt is rising, reaching $215,000 (Education Data).

The decision to become a generalist or specialist can be difficult. Selection of which training to enter is not only financially-driven but also relates to one's interests and lifestyle goals. Primary care can sometimes allow increased flexibility in finding a job and choosing a schedule. Specialists are less abundant, which may place a greater demand on their time. Nevertheless, primary care physicians have among the highest rates of burnout— hovering around 55% in 2017. Common concerns cited were the ever-growing influx of bureaucratic tasks from the EHR and the longer hours (Medscape, 2017).

Yet, in systems where primary care support is solid, patient outcomes are better, particularly in resource-poor settings. For instance, several studies showed lower levels of all-cause mortality in post-neonates and patients with stroke, heart disease, and cancer, hearkening to the importance of preventive screening (Starfield, 2005).

With the growing gap in primary care, patients may increasingly find it difficult to see their PCPs and instead access urgent care clinics or emergency departments. What would be the outcome of having multiple physicians involved in patient care? What are some of the responsibilities of a generalist and a specialist? Do too many cooks spoil the broth?

Case 8: "Just Need a Refill of My Prescriptions"

A thirty-five-year-old patient came into the clinic as a new patient visit. He thought he had a straightforward request for his new doctor: three medication refills. He was on albuterol for his asthma, omeprazole for gastroesophageal reflux, and sertraline for depression.

A dive into his history revealed that his father had had a heart attack in his late forties. The patient also reported enjoying a "good old American habit" of drinking beer nightly, sometimes four to six cans. He did not seem aware that this amount could contribute to all his health issues. He was surprised and defensive when I asked him further about it. I pointed out that not addressing the alcohol problem, which qualified as alcohol dependence, would be like putting out a fire while there is still a gas leak.

On a second visit, he brought his girlfriend for support. We performed a health assessment, blood pressure check, and reviewed his lab results — all of which were acceptable. He asked about his cholesterol level, which showed an elevated LDL, or "bad cholesterol." He noticed that the LDL was elevated and wondered if it was time for him to consider starting a "statin[23]." His blood pressure was a little high, but he was also overweight. As I reviewed his medications and assessed the risks and benefits of starting a new drug, I asked him to consider reducing his alcohol intake.

His partner was also concerned about the harm caused by his heavy alcohol intake. He scolded her and then defensively responded to me, "How come you bring this up each visit?" He could not or would not accept responsibility or acknowledge that his dependence was an obstacle to his optimal health, including mental health. Maybe he reasoned that his health risks, including heart disease, were a result of fate rather than behavior. He rationalized in his mind that medications would provide him a pathway to health, even while his habits were stoking the flames of disease.

Case 9: Multiple Episodes of Pneumonia on Chemotherapy

I cared for a 58-year-old female diagnosed with lymphoma, a type of cancer in the lymphatic system that can sometimes be difficult to diagnose. She developed fatigue and gastro-intestinal upset for months. After several doctor visits, lab investigations showed mild anemia and elevated liver function tests. A CT scan showed thickening in the esophagus with multiple lymph nodes surrounding it. The GI doctor performed an endoscopic ultrasound with a biopsy that confirmed non-Hodgkin's lymphoma.

On the cancer diagnosis day, she came in for ongoing fatigue. She was upset that there was a delay in the diagnosis after informing physicians that she had felt fatigued for months. She was grateful to know that it was not just in her head. She was referred to an oncologist to discuss treatment options.

She met with an oncologist, began chemotherapy, and came in for a check-up. One of the medications was Rituxan (rituximab) combined with other agents. Rituxan is a monoclonal antibody that binds to a receptor on B-cells (CD20), triggering a flurry of inflammatory mediators. The therapy leads to complement- and antibody-mediated destruction of affected cells (Cerny, 2002). She had started the treatment and felt that she was tolerating it.

About one month later, she returned to my clinic. She informed me that her oncologist started her on antibiotics because she had developed a dry cough and fever. The chest radiograph was worrisome for pneumonia. I asked her to take an inhaler with a steroid and another medication while she completed the course of antibiotics. She had not developed any untoward symptoms of chemotherapy up to this point. Still, I wondered if we needed to consider another explanation since she never really had any change in her status other than the cough.

A couple of weeks later, she reported that her oncologist had given her another antibiotic. I reviewed her chest x-rays and noted findings described as a "ground-glass" appearance on the lung CT scan. I wondered about different infections[24] in her immunocompromised state. I reviewed her medications and reminded myself of a patient I had seen in my fellowship training. He had been given Rituxan (Rituximab) and developed an acute pneumonia picture. My concern was that the process was causally related to the therapy.

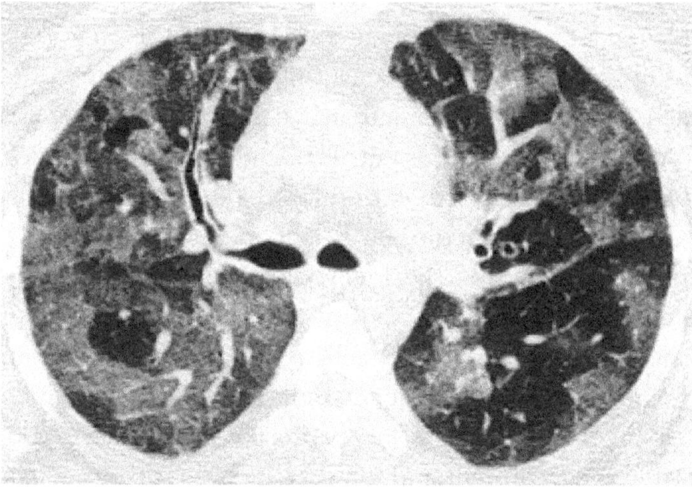

Figure 1: The CT scan of the thorax shows an example of patchy ground-glass changes. Source: Creative Commons.

I reviewed rituximab-induced interstitial lung disease (Wagner, 2007). This condition usually occurs after one month of therapy and causes breathlessness, fever, and a dry, non-productive cough. This diagnosis could wholly explain the symptoms she was experiencing. I reached out to the oncologist and left a message about my concerns. He returned my call and agreed with this consideration. Since this process could worsen, I started her on high-dose steroids and scheduled her in the clinic weekly for the course of treatment. I observed her significant improvement with the therapy during the subsequent weeks.

Case 10: Having the Heart to Prescribe

Some years ago, a patient was concerned about her increased anxiety. Her husband experienced challenges with chronic illnesses, and she had increased stress as his sole caregiver She asked me if there was any medication that I could prescribe her to help. I emphasized that it would benefit her to take time off each day and look for other sources of support. For instance, her husband's doctor could arrange for a visiting nurse or home health physical therapy to offload the responsibility. I told her that I did not feel there was any role for additional medications. She was already taking a select serotonin-reuptake inhibitor (SSRI). I did not think that a benzodiazepine, which she asked for specifically, would provide any additional support in her predicament.

A hospital report came in for my review a week after we met. The patient was hospitalized for vague chest pain and nonspecific findings on her ECG. She underwent a cardiac catheterization, which did not demonstrate any significant blockages requiring intervention. She was under the care of a cardiologist and followed up with him in his clinic one week later. Per his report, her chest pain had improved, and he thought stress was a factor. It went away after the cardiologist gave her a dose of a sedative.

She returned to my clinic for a follow-up visit. She was complaining of increased stress. The cardiologist prescribed her lorazepam, a short-acting benzo, recommending that she "take one tablet (2mg) every 8 hours as *needed* for anxiety." He gave her enough to last a few weeks if taken every 8 hours. And since she was feeling anxious after the medication wore off, that was how she took it. After several days of benefit, she noticed that the dose did not help as much. Her anxiety was peaking again. She was tearful and pleaded with me to renew the prescription and increase the amount. As I listened to her concerns and acknowledged them, I realized her request put me outside my comfort zone for managing anxiety.

I stepped out of the room and collected my thoughts in my office. I often do this because it gives me a chance to prepare a clear message and review the chart before I return to discuss my recommendations with the patient. The notes from the cardiologist who saw her confirmed that he prescribed forty tablets of lorazepam. It was late Friday afternoon, and I could not help but think the following: *Since when does a cardiologist write anti-anxiety medicine! He dug this hole; maybe he should dig himself out of it.*

Benzodiazepine Overdose

Benzodiazepines are one of the most frequently prescribed drugs in the United States. Any substance that dissolves pain or panic is a double-edged sword. In both the field of psychiatry and on the street, their value in treating anxiety and potential for addiction was no secret.

Benzodiazepines continue to make the headlines: the FDA estimates ninety-two million prescriptions were written in the US in 2019. Fifty percent of the patients took them for two months or longer (Safai, 2020). The number of people dying from benzodiazepine overdose increased from 1,135 to 9,711 over 20 years (1999 to 2019). Many of these deaths were in people who also took opiates, mainly fentanyl (NIDA) .

A few years before seeing the patient in Case 10, I had discovered that a patient I had seen overdosed on benzodiazepines. Despite my recommendations to maintain the same dose (she received the prescription from another doctor), she used her spouse's medicine and her allotment. Her father-in-law, also a patient of mine, informed me that the paramedics found her "blue" from respiratory arrest, and they could not revive her.

I rehearsed what I would say to the patient before returning to the exam room, taking a deep breath before opening the door. I informed her of my concern that the lorazepam may be causing more of a problem than helping. She described an escalation of anxiety, even in the setting of taking it "around-the-clock," suggesting tolerance. Although it is often a result of long-term use, tolerance can develop in as little as days to weeks (Ashton, 2005). It was realistic to consider that her routine use of short-acting benzodiazepines may have intensified her anxiety.

Unfortunately, she would need to taper off meds while working on beneficial coping strategies with a therapist. It can sometimes be challenging to ensure self-care needs are met while caring for a spouse or other loved one. Caregiving can be a stressor and provoke anxiety, but a person can learn to set boundaries. Medications do not nullify stressors, and she might need further assistance, such as a counselor or psychiatrist.

She expressed fear of reducing her medications because the anxiety was only worsening. I provided her with guidance on tapering and consoled her as she reacted to this news. She could contact the prescribing doctor for any future prescriptions.

I spoke with the cardiologist to express my concerns. He was surprised that she took the medication every 8 hours and agreed with the plan. Prescribing this added more work for him and more anxiety for her. I reasoned with him that, even though he showed compassion for the patient, consulting with her primary care doctor would have allowed a hand-off of an issue outside his purview.

Generalist and Specialist: Two Sides of the Same Coin

The Generalist Enhances Care

The job requirements include being a skilled clinician, care coordinator, and collaborator. Whether a physician, physician assistant, or nurse practitioner, a generalist provides a patient with a vital access point to healthcare. A solid clinician-patient relationship flourishes over time. Unlike the ER or urgent care, patients forge partnerships with one primary care provider, strengthening their medical care.

"I like that you know my history, concerns, and goals" is a common sentiment expressed by longstanding patients. A physician develops a rapport with a patient, enabling them to earnestly discuss their health concerns with a physician who is aware of their prior medical history, habits, and individual challenges. A doctor-patient relationship can be an impetus for a patient to overcome obstacles and make behavior change possible. Patients often have a rift between their chronic disease(s) and an instigating behavior— not routinely explored in clinic visits. Sometimes that void gets filled with medications rather than attention. Within this web of interaction, a primary care physician may start to engage with a patient to expose the trigger, the history that set the behavior in motion.

A PCP is a forest-for-the-trees-specialist—a "generalist-specialist." The years of post-graduate training for an internist (3) and family practitioner (4) allow ample time to develop a rubric by which a physician may address any medical concern. The emphasis is on the breadth of knowledge over depth. A longitudinal relationship with a patient provides a whole-patient approach. It is typical for a patient to schedule an appointment with their PCP to review the specialist's recommendations before starting treatment. Not only do patients want to keep the PCP informed, but they also want them to weigh in on the treatment plan.

For this reason, I was able to screen the patient in **Case 9** and identify potential toxicity from her therapy. The patient had not initially realized that it could have been a side effect of the medications. She also had trouble seeing her busy specialist even as she deteriorated. After reviewing the symptoms, the chest x-ray, and her history, medication side effects needed consideration. She had a preponderance of symptoms without a clear set of infections. There was a chance for early recognition of a potentially life-threatening condition.

The Generalist Strategizes and Monitors Prescribing

One type of clinic visit is an appointment for medication renewal. It allows a physician and patient to discuss each medication's indications, risks, and benefits. As in **Case 8**, a PCP is not a reflexive prescriber who renews prescriptions without reviewing the patient's health history. They do not write pain or sleep medications without exploring deeper into the condition's causes and expectations of treatment. A physician must walk a narrow line of being a collaborator rather than an enabler to someone's harmful behaviors, including a growing medication list.

One way to look at disease is the body's adaptation to a pressure exerted by some imbalance. Chronic diseases emerge when there is a multi-system imbalance. For instance, individuals that are overweight may develop insulin resistance and impaired function until they can no longer effectively manage blood sugar and develop diabetes. Many conditions are interrelated, even though doctors sometimes treat each condition separately with different medicines.

However, most medications that treat chronic diseases do not offer a cure. Instead, they may mitigate risk, a form of secondary prevention. It also does not mean that primary prevention measures are exhausted. We often ascribe a medication's "main effects" to those effects that reduce the severity of a condition. But by exerting any pressure on the body, they create a degree of imbalance, or "side effect," in how the body copes. No medication guarantees the level of health that eating a natural diet and keeping an active lifestyle do. As a physician, there is no greater joy than providing health empowerment and seeing patients improve without medications.

General practitioners treat an increasing population of geriatric patients and other medically complex patients on multiple medications. Geriatricians and internists who have additional training on the specific issues encountered in the elderly are in short supply. Along with advancing age comes chronic diseases, more treatment options, and more referrals to specialists. In one study of seniors with a mean age of 76.9 years, 40.6% used multiple medications, and 35.6% had polypharmacy, defined as more than five prescribed medications (Golchin, 2015).

With medications, more is not better. It is usually worse. Patients on more medications have harmful side effects that contribute to an increased risk of falls and hospitalizations (Leipzig, 1999; CIH, 2016). Physicians should discuss the potential harms and benefits of medications and inform their patients regarding these. Studies suggest that 1 in 9 emergency department visits are related to some form of an adverse event from a pill, most of them either moderate (74.6%) or severe (9.8%) (Zed, 2008). These adverse events account for an estimated 17 million emergency department visits and 8.7 million hospitalizations in the United States annually (Johnson, 1995).

Should doctors limit the number of medications prescribed to each patient? One of a physician's jobs is to determine when there is a time to "do no harm" and avoid drugs or to prescribe the lowest effective dose. Just because a patient has a treatable process like neck muscle tension does not mean they need medication. They may be straining themselves as they sit in front of a computer screen for hours authoring a book. Health concerns are like the body calling on the brain to understand the why and how. The root cause approach is practical and can sometimes be therapeutic, i.e., by stopping harmful side effects. Some patients achieve significant benefits by tapering or stopping unhelpful medications if nonpharmacologic treatments are an option (Scott, 2015).

Every clinic visit provides an opportunity for the physician and patient to discuss the following criteria: each medication's purpose, prescriber, risks, and benefits. All drugs have side effects and interactions; some may even be more harmful than helpful. A physician can create a priority list for a patient's medications and consider which may be stopped or reduced. Several online resources, such as the Beers criteria, Epocrates, and Medstopper, can alert a physician and patient to consider deprescribing[25] a medication (Halli-Tierney, 2019). Additionally, electronic health records include programs that reduce polypharmacy and cross-check for potential drug interactions.

When I worked as a primary care doctor, my patients came in at least yearly with all their medications brought in a bag for review.[26] I was astonished by the frequency of duplicate bottles, potentially harmful over-the-counter medications, and "as-needed" medications accumulating over the year from several prescribers. I reviewed the criteria for each drug. If a patient took meds infrequently, had little benefit, or had a high risk for side effects, I coordinated a taper or stop plan with the patient and discussed it with the prescribing specialist, if any.

I placed the duplicates or discontinued bottles into a red protected-information waste bag in front of their eyes. Patients often expressed concern about this, wondering if it was OK to stop a long-term medication or a prior doctor's prescriptions. Usually after reassurance that I will monitor their health closely, they felt relieved as I threw out the medications. Frequently, patients returned to the clinic feeling much better, recognizing that the pills had been causing side effects.

The Generalist can Mitigate Harm

Multiple prescribers lead to polypharmacy and drug interactions. Specialists often add to a patient's prescriptions list. Someone with chronic disease usually has overlapping conditions, like obesity, high blood pressure, diabetes, lipid problems, gastroesophageal reflux, and gout. Someone with obesity could easily receive five or more medications from different specialists.

The Generalist Focuses on the Big Picture, not only on Specific Therapies

Primary care doctors significantly contribute to the review of prescribed medications and their interactions. Certain medicines that generalists do not routinely prescribe fall under a specialist's purview. These include medications for heart failure, rheumatoid arthritis, psoriasis, Crohn's disease, and cancer.

A specialist may not be able to review a patient's complete health history or have access to their medication list. It was not uncommon for me as a specialist to see a patient in the clinic for an infectious diseases concern before we received any records. When more physicians are involved in a patient's care, hyper-focused care is more likely, often without tackling the disease's behavioral aspects and risk factors. This is detrimental to the patient. The PCP serves as the quarterback for the patient's treatment plan.

The Generalist is More Familiar with a Patient's Longitudinal Medical History and Risks

A solid doctor-patient relationship enables a doctor to understand a patient's background and risk factors. Patients may report to urgent care or emergency care doctors for acute needs, such as a patient with asthma and kidney disease developing a viral infection. Without detailed records of a person's history or an appropriate setting to discuss health risk factors, sometimes a doctor treats a patient with a "just-in-case" approach or medicates them without knowledge of underlying health issues. Even short-term treatment can have risks. For example, doctors may need to reduce the medication dose or frequency, including antibiotics, in patients with kidney or liver problems. These oversights could result in harmful side effects and drug interactions.

The Specialist Focuses and Collaborates

Specialists serve four roles in healthcare: 1) they provide a patient and physician with another opportunity to review the history and physical findings and determine the potential cause and work up from a focused point of view; 2) they have more experience in the diagnosis of diseases in that specific discipline; 3) they can provide the patient with more detailed treatment recommendations and education; 4) they perform procedures specific to that discipline.

The premise behind specialty training is to expand a physician's experience in one area of interest. More than twenty-two approved subspecialties in the specialty of internal medicine exist, requiring from one to three years of additional training. Focused time equips a physician with a more significant knowledge base and diagnostic insight into one system or discipline. A more extensive background reduces the gap of uncertainty or, at least, strengthens the skillset to address it.

Certain specialties include training in system-specific procedures. Whether it is a colonoscopy or EGD[27] for a gastroenterologist (GI) or a bronchoscopy for a pulmonologist, the instruments bring a specialist closer to the source of the disease. They can take samples for a pathologist to inspect the tissues under microscopy corresponding to a patient's signs and symptoms.

Studies support that specialist involvement improves patient care for some conditions. For instance, a cardiologist enhances a patient's treatment of congestive heart failure; psychiatrists improve care for someone with depression; in patients with HIV or endocarditis, infectious diseases specialists enhance patient outcomes (Donohoe, 1998; Landon, 2005).

All specialists must remember that they are consultants for the referring physician and the patient. Without a physician's trust in referring a patient, the specialist would not have a job. During my fellowship, my mentor in infectious diseases would remind me of the "three A's" of specialty medicine: a specialist should be able, available, and affable. The overarching goal is to enhance patient care while improving the quality of experience for each physician involved.

On My Decision to Become a Specialist

I had a challenging time deciding to pursue specialty training. I wondered if being a specialist would decrease my flexibility because of less job availability. Would the doctor-patient relationship I enjoyed during residency be limited because of only seeing someone for focused issues? In college, I developed interests that dated back to my childhood—infectious diseases, microbiology, and tropical medicine. It seemed like I would be a good fit for a specialization in infectious diseases.

After my internal medicine residency, I committed to taking the two additional years of training to become a specialist in infectious diseases. I entered a discipline that supported a comprehensive assessment, gave me a chance to collaborate with colleagues across disciplines, and provided me with a skillset to assist patients when they are ill. In actuality, the starting point for a specialist is the same as a generalist: prioritizing connecting with the patient and understanding their concerns.

Specializing as an Infectious Diseases (ID) Specialist

The Infectious Diseases fellowship spans two to three additional years of post-graduate training after internal medicine residency. Upon completion of the program, an ID specialist may work in the clinical setting, perform research, and teach in an academic fellowship and residency program. Additional job opportunities include working in the pharmaceutical industry, global health, as a hospital epidemiologist (IDSA website).

A clinical ID specialist gains skills in evaluating patients with complex presentations, interpreting health information, and developing a work-up and treatment strategy. Information gathering is an essential part in the discipline. A physician may have a lengthy visit with a patient, review documentation and historical records, and then speak to family members and caregivers. The objective is to garner information on what really occurred and offer insight into what caused a change from a person's usual state of health.

The Specialist Benefits from a Holistic View

A specialist develops proficiency in a specific area of health after additional training. Consultants may seemingly conjure up rare diagnoses in their field and gain a more accurate perspective of what the patient is experiencing. However, a specialist enters the thought process and the formation of a diagnosis the same way as a generalist— through careful discussion with the patient and a thorough physical examination. When faced with uncertainty, a specialist must not abandon the general assessment of a patient's concern, rooted in collaboration, active communication, and empathic listening.

Abraham Maslow said, "If the only tool you have is a hammer, you tend to treat everything as if it were a nail." The words resonate when a specialist approaches a patient— they should not forget to interpret the symptoms that a patient presents with a broad scope before narrowing the focus.

There are, in truth, no specialties in medicine, since to know fully many of the most important diseases, a [person] must be familiar with their manifestations in many organs.
—Sir William Osler

Summary: Generalist and Specialist

Generalist

- Broad knowledge base and sees the big picture
- Strategizes and monitors prescribing
- Can mitigate harm and address behaviors
- More familiar with longitudinal history

Specialist

- Focused knowledge and heuristics
- Performs procedures in the discipline
- Bridge between physician and patient for education, management, and second opinion

CHAPTER 6

On the Difficult Diagnosis and Sudden Health Changes

A condition such as a stroke or a heart attack reminds us that, although we measure our lives in years, some of the most significant life changes can occur in a matter of seconds.

Key Points

- All physicians face situations where they cannot determine a diagnosis with the information provided. As the disease smolders, a diagnosis may begin to surface.

- Approaching a difficult diagnosis requires close collaboration with the patient, including developing a plan as to timing, course of action, and monitoring.

- Some conditions present a narrow window of stability and then deteriorate rapidly, requiring collaborative effort for identification and stabilization.

Cases

Case 11: Mononucleosis Syndrome

Case 12: TB or not TB?

Case 13: Blood Breakdown after a Stem Cell Transplant

Case 14: "I Thought I saw Blood!"

Case 15: The Last Bleed

Case 16: A Stroke of Misfortune

Case 17: When a Visitor Becomes a Patient

The practice of medicine comes with some degree of uncertainty. A diagnosis may not materialize like a description in a textbook. Furthermore, even many hours of formal training cannot guarantee that a physician will see various disease manifestations. Uncertainty can be a source of medical errors, harm, unnecessary testing, more hospitalizations and referrals, and increased stress. The chapter explores two significant diagnostic challenges physicians encounter: complex diagnoses and sudden changes. A sensitivity to these themes can prepare a doctor to develop a method that addresses and embraces uncertainty.

The Difficult Diagnosis: The Snowball in the Blizzard

Steve Hatch, MD, uses the metaphor "Snowball in a Blizzard" as the title of his book to describe the difficulty of finding an abnormality in a background of noise (Hatch, 2016). He mentions the example of a radiologist trying to find a tumor on a mammogram, which can be incredibly challenging amid a milieu of dense breast tissue. Every physician faces similar uncertainty as they approach difficult diagnoses. In one study of 848 physician surveys, 50% of physicians reported that it happened in more than 5% of patient presentations (Sarkar, 2013). Even though the report was from experienced physicians, they cited inadequate knowledge base and challenges with interpretation of information as the primary reasons.

There are myriad general concerns, such as chest pain, gastric pain, fatigue, aches, dizziness, and weakness, which do not fit easily into one diagnosis. Compounding a patient's presentation is the interaction of the brain on the condition— one in which the biomedical model[28] is often shortsighted. A person interprets somatic[29] complaints with a mental narrative, which is a response to feeling unwell and can itself affect the process. Additionally, mental distress can lead to physical complaints or somatization. In a study of somaticizing patients in a primary care setting, as many as 83% had conditions such as anxiety and depression (Aiarzaguena, 2008). Nevertheless, it is a disservice for a doctor to conclude that a complaint emanates just from a patient's mind and stop searching.

A critical starting point is to regard every patient's concern as legitimate. A patient may sense that their health is not right, but a physician cannot zero in on a diagnosis without enough evidence. Sometimes unknowingly, a physician finds themselves in the middle of a diagnostic challenge, where continued efforts are not producing answers for their patients. A primary care physician may suggest a referral to a specialist, but if the process is not apparent, it is hard to know which one. In the meantime, physicians must develop a plan with the patient, involving options and contingencies while the problem withers away or intensifies.

How does a physician assist a patient with a difficult diagnosis?

They approach it the same way as any health concern. The reason for a patient's troubles may not be easy to discover, and it is not necessarily because the doctor is not competent or knowledgeable enough. Sometimes an illness may not manifest typically. A host of symptoms does not always clarify things if they are all nonspecific.

Indeed, there is a sweet spot in arriving at a diagnosis. There may be no harm in watchful waiting,[30] allowing symptoms to develop enough to justify further testing. A little waiting may provide enough time for a disease to show up on a CT scan or bloodwork. However, waiting too long holds up therapy and can expose a person to discomfort or risk.

The cornerstone of any diagnosis is a thorough, open interview. What is paramount are the words a patient uses to describe a concern and the clarifying questions a physician asks. Listening to understand while being sensitive to bias is crucial to detecting a cause. Imagine guessing a puzzle's image with missing pieces. When there are fewer pieces in the picture, there is a lower likelihood of making an accurate prediction. A carefully conducted interview can fill in those empty spaces. Nevertheless, not all diagnoses come after one visit or several, for that matter.

A disease process can take time to present, grow, and enable a safe way to diagnose it. When the disease occurs in deeper vessels and the lymphatic system, often the manifestations are nonspecific, including the results of the blood and radiologic tests. Since many infections can present similarly, a shot-gun approach is not always high-yield, cost-effective, or worry-free[31]. A physician must balance considering the most likely possibilities with discerning when it may be time to search for unusual causes.

After carefully examining the skin, the body's largest organ, some complex diagnoses come to fruition. The skin houses a network of vessels that mirror what is going on throughout the entire body. Occasionally, diseases can present on the skin, facilitating a diagnosis with less invasive measures, such as a punch biopsy. Examples of systemic diseases with skin findings include sarcoidosis, T-cell lymphoma, malignant melanoma, and metastatic squamous cell carcinoma of the lungs.

A Difficult Diagnosis May Fit a Pattern that an Astute Physician Detects

In medicine, seldom is a condition diagnosed on the spot. However, it can happen if a doctor identifies a pattern. An astute physician can invoke a diagnosis like a magician conjuring up a spell. While rounding with us on a particularly vexing patient, one of my infectious disease mentors did just that. The patient had lip ulcers and a generalized rash, and some on his palm that looked like targets. He examined the patient and gave him the diagnosis right away. I remember when my mentor told the patient that he had "Mycoplasma with erythema multiforme," as if putting the disease in its place. He did have the chest X-ray findings seen in Mycoplasma, the cause of "walking pneumonia," and all his tests, including HIV and syphilis, were normal. We were spellbound as we reviewed this uncommon presentation.

Case 11: Mononucleosis Syndrome

A fifty-six-year-old female developed multiple concerns: weakness, chills, and jaundice. She had difficulty pinpointing the sequence of the symptoms, a dilemma not so uncommon when an illness develops gradually. An exam did not show any swollen lymph nodes or pharyngitis but did reveal jaundice and fullness of her liver. Indeed, she was ill enough to require hospitalization.

The team performed numerous tests for infectious diseases, but none singled out the process. The monospot,[32] Epstein Barr Virus (EBV), and Cytomegalovirus (CMV) titers were negative. A CT scan showed an enlarged liver and spleen. Over a week, she improved to the point that she could go home without a diagnosis. The series of findings suggested a typhoidal **mononucleosis syndrome (Table 2)**.

Table 2: Causes of Mononucleosis-Like Syndrome
Epstein Barr Virus (EBV) ~90%
Adenovirus
Cytomegalovirus (CMV)
Toxoplasmosis (*Toxoplasma gondii*)
Human Immunodeficiency Virus (HIV) – Acute retroviral syndrome from HIV
Hepatitis A, B, C
Herpes Simplex Virus (HSV) – Primary disease
Human Herpesvirus 6 (HHV-6)
Rubella virus
Strep throat (Group A Strep)
Noninfectious Causes

A sore throat, fever, and neck lymph node swelling characterize the classic mononucleosis syndrome. EBV infection is the most common cause. However, a more systemic process, or typhoidal[33] presentation, is a less frequent manifestation of EBV. Patients with this syndrome present with fevers, fatigue, and an enlarged spleen and liver. It is a type of presentation that is one of the most mysterious ways a disease manifests in the body.

Many conditions fall in this bucket (**Table 3**), making it frequently challenging to pinpoint a diagnosis (Hurt, 2007). Nonspecific test results are typical: liver tests may be high, suggesting hepatitis; the white blood cells and platelet counts might be low because of an enlarged spleen. There is often not enough information to confirm a diagnosis. Of particular concern was lymphoma, a type of lymph node cancer. Because some of these conditions improve on their own, the dilemma becomes to wait or not wait to get more information, such as a liver biopsy.

She reported that her fever and fatigue still did not resolve during a three-week follow-up. It was not clear that she was going to improve on her own. We sought clarification with a liver biopsy. Unfortunately, her results indicated a process that could have many potential causes. Biopsies can only tell how a condition affects the tissue at a cellular level. It does not always declare a diagnosis.

The pathologist wondered about hemophagocytic lymphohistiocytosis (HLH), a rare inflammatory condition caused by an autoimmune reaction, cancer, or an infection (Griffin, 2020). We discussed the results. There were no findings that could pinpoint a cause. It was like taking a step forward to nowhere. I brought up with her a strategy to address this diagnostic challenge. Fortunately, she felt better, although the process's trigger remained unidentified.

Case 12: TB or not TB?

A patient from East Africa presented with peritoneal fluid, lymph nodes, and peritoneal lining thickening. The pathology showed non-caseating granulomas, a feature associated with sarcoidosis but not exclusively. The exact cause of this inflammatory condition remains unclear. The immune system recruits white blood cells to tissues, similar to how it responds to bacteria, viruses, or other particles. If you look up "sarcoidosis" and "Ethiopia," you will find articles published on how this rare condition resembles more prevalent diseases in the country like tuberculosis.

I reminded myself to think of horses, not zebras — or, in this case, was it the other way around? Sometimes infections like tuberculosis can form these types of granulomas. The patient's blood test (QuantiFERON) was positive for tuberculosis. Still, it was not clear if it was a latent infection plus sarcoidosis or if this was all a manifestation of active tuberculosis.

I saw her in my hospital a few days after she was discharged from another local hospital. There she had an additional peritoneal biopsy. I talked to the pathologist and alerted him that I found her case worrisome for tuberculosis. He informed me that he had already looked at the smears[34] and did not find anything. My call was enough to get him to look again. Sometimes seeing the bacillus that causes tuberculosis can be like finding a needle in a haystack.

He called me just hours later, saying that he saw one acid-fast bacillus. The lab sent the samples for culture and sensitivity confirmation, which can take eight weeks. However, there was enough indication to start the patient on the four-drug tuberculosis regimen[35]. After about one week, she already felt much better.

She had peritoneal tuberculosis. None of the cultures grew; no genetic tests were ever positive. Yet, tuberculosis is challenging to grow in the lab from patients with this type of TB. References cite only 20% of the time are cultures positive (Debi, 2014).

Case 13: Blood Breakdown in a Patient after a Stem Cell Transplant

As an infectious disease fellow, our program in Washington, DC, collaborated with the National Institutes of Health (NIH) in Bethesda, Maryland. This center offered fellows an opportunity to gain experience at a major referral center for the east coast. I met a patient after ordering the correct test to confirm her diagnosis.

It was common during the daily rounds that infectious diseases and Hematology/Oncology[36] fellows would talk about patient cases collaboratively and decide upon future consults. It was something I enjoyed. One of the fellows brought up a vexing case of a patient who had sickle cell anemia but underwent a stem cell transplant with a good result. Sickle cell is a condition where a specific type of hemoglobin (Hemoglobin S) causes the red blood cells to be misshapen, break down easily (hemolysis), and impede small vessel blood flow. The blockages prevent oxygen from transmitting to tissues and lead to cellular injury or death. Patients may experience substantial pain and other complications from a sickle cell crisis. Excessive blood transfusions can cause some patients with sickle cell anemia to have a condition of iron overload known as hemochromatosis, aided by therapeutic blood withdrawal.

The same problems occurred with the patient that the oncology fellow and I discussed on rounds. She was a 21-year-old from Puerto Rico who had received a stem cell transplant, a procedure where doctors give healthy bone marrow cells to overtake the production of sickle cells. The patient's procedure was a success, and, by all accounts, there was a complete cure.

Yet, months after the transplant, she developed a fever that would not go away. She also had headaches, neck pain, fatigue, and joint aches. She was on an antibiotic (Bactrim) to prevent her from getting a particular type of fungal infection known as *Pneumocystis jirovecii* pneumonia (PJP) after receiving steroids for the transplant. She saw a doctor who thought she had a sinus infection and prescribed her levofloxacin, which led to temporary improvement. She came to the NIH after bloodwork revealed that she was somehow losing blood the same way she had with sickle cell before— through breakdown.[37]

The oncology team evaluated her and performed a battery of tests. The bloodwork results suggested that she had a return of her sickle cell disease. However, the bone marrow biopsy did not show any concerns that she was relapsing. The fellow asked me if I thought it was an infection. I reminded myself about the conditions that lead to blood breakdown. The one that I was concerned about was malaria. There has not been a malaria case in Puerto Rico since the 1950s, but I half-jokingly requested her to check a malaria smear.

A few days later, despite all the tests, including a Computed Tomography of the abdomen and pelvis, we were no closer to determining the cause of her fever. However, the patient did have a large spleen, not an uncommon finding in any condition that leads to blood breakdown, including sickle cell disease. After the spleen deals with years of blood breakdown, it gradually wears down, not unlike someone who had their spleen removed.[38] A dysfunctional or absent spleen leads to an increased risk of more severe infections, including malaria, babesiosis, *Capnocytophaga canimorsus*,[39] from dog bites, and diseases from bacteria for which we have vaccines: *Neisseria meningitidis*, *Streptococcus pneumoniae*, and *Haemophilus influenza*.

We discussed the patient's issues yet again days later. Nothing had improved. I recommended adding a peripheral blood smear. The best way to look for parasites in red blood cells is to take a blood sample and examine the cells under a microscope. If we did not perform the test, we could miss something. By then, about five days into her hospitalization, it was clear that we needed to check this.

The fellow called me from the lab about an hour after I spoke with her. The patient had a positive smear. We all went downstairs to review the slides. There were tiny ring-shaped parasites in the red blood cells. There were multiple forms— some of which had a cross-like appearance (Maltese cross). We speculated about the worst form of malaria *Plasmodium falciparum*, but we convinced ourselves with the parasitologist attending present that it could not be malaria: her parasite load would have been fatal.

After putting things together and realizing that she had multiple blood transfusions, we wondered if she may have acquired the parasite *Babesia microti* from this route. It is known for its prevalence in Massachusetts as a tick-borne infection, and some serologic surveys of blood donors from the state indicate a prevalence rate of 3-5% (Levin, 2017).

In 2008, the FDA reported that *Babesia* was the most frequent pathogen contaminating blood transfusions in the US. Presumably, that is what happened to this patient. She had not visited an endemic area. An inquiry of her blood donors revealed that one of her seventeen blood product donors had a high titer for *Babesia*, though genomic testing could not corroborate this.[40] She received the blood product a week before her transplant. The patient's splenic dysfunction and the steroids made her incapable of clearing the infection. It can be difficult to eradicate even with treatment in this setting.

It was a privilege to meet the patient to provide her with a precise diagnosis for a challenging condition. The patient was relieved, her fever responded after two days of treatment, and the other symptoms improved gradually. All teams collaborated on a case write-up to raise awareness of this condition (Cirino, 2008). It is still one of the most successful reminders in my career of the importance of revisiting the presentation and identifying practical ways to investigate a person's concerns.

Approaching Challenging Diagnoses

A vague, confusing presentation can increase a doctor's concern about missing something. It can even make a physician wonder whether they are skilled enough to find the cause. In patients with cancer, 20 percent report to their primary care doctor with key symptoms three or more times before a referral to an oncologist (Lyratzopolous, 2014). Early diagnosis of cancer is crucial but challenging. In pancreatic cancer, the difference in the five-year survival rate between localized disease and metastasis is 37.4% compared to 2.9%, respectively. Specific diagnoses like cancer present slowly, nonspecifically, and are more challenging to diagnose.

Hovering over every physician in these circumstances is the concern of malpractice. A failure to diagnose or a delayed diagnosis comprises 39 percent of medical malpractice lawsuit claims. There is a point when the nonspecific, mild symptoms start to escalate to more specific, acute symptoms. Ideally, the time to diagnose is before a disease can cause a threat to health or become harder to treat.

Fortunately, there are crucial ways to address challenging diagnoses for patients and doctors alike. Here are five suggestions to approach these dilemmas:

- **Go Back to the History and Physical Exam**

History and exams are one of the physician's most essential tools. A dying art in the era of advanced medical technology, a good history can still assist significantly in arriving at a diagnosis; from some estimates, 70 to 90 percent of the time. Whenever I face a diagnostic challenge, I go back to the patient and listen again to their words, determining the evolution of their symptoms.

A follow-up physical examination while reviewing history is critical. The best exam includes a follow-up visit. The patient may have had a chance to think about the symptoms or questions more, the process may have developed, the exam may change, or a physician may have missed a finding on the prior exam. Like any skill, a physician's clinical intuition combines knowledge, experience, and dynamic prediction through close observation.

- **Keep Open Communication**

It is vital to keep the channels open to discuss any questions or concerns, even if they may not seem immediately relevant. I like to reassure the patient that I will continue to search for answers and that I am "stubborn" on their behalf. The person can contact me to update me on their status between visits. I usually keep visits at monthly intervals to review a patient's progress.

• Go toward the place where there is the most notable change.

Patients may develop localizing symptoms, for instance, right lower quadrant abdominal pain. After performing a thorough examination of all systems that may overlap in one area, screening blood tests and targeted studies may be helpful. Laboratory tests can change over time with a developing process, so it is essential to look for trends in the white blood count, the red blood count, or liver tests. Doctors can order an imaging test such as a CT scan or ultrasound for a localizable concern. Where one encounters an abnormality in studies, more invasive tests may assist in the diagnosis. It often requires getting closer to the problems with a scope or a sample guided by interventional radiology. As Carl Sagan stated, the key point is that "the absence of evidence is not always evidence of absence." Remember, every patient is experiencing a valid concern.

• Watchful waiting requires a commitment to diligence from doctors and patients.

Nonspecific symptoms cannot always help a physician

discern disease severity. For example, pancreatic cancer can take months to diagnose because patients start with nonspecific abdominal pain. Watchful waiting requires careful planning and goal setting. If a person is not suffering from severe symptoms, they may be safe enough to monitor over time. It is helpful for the doctor to see the patient frequently and consider the utility of additional testing, such as an imaging study or diagnostic test.

- **Consider collaborative discussions and a referral for a second opinion.**

There will always be knowledge gaps with the ever-increasing amount of medical literature. I used to think that being a specialist, I would have a more confined and manageable knowledge foundation than a generalist. I thought wrong. It is just as complex and ever-developing. Remember the COVID-19 example in chapter 2. There are more publications than there is time to review them.

It is not unusual for multiple providers to be aware of a patient's health issues. Hospitalists often take turns covering patients. There is a sign-out and transfer of care from provider to provider. It can offer a jumping-off point for collaboration and problem-solving.

It would be a disservice to the patient not to collaborate with colleagues. I find it helpful and exciting to walk down to the radiology reading rooms to see the studies with the radiologists, check the slides myself in the lab, review the biopsies with a pathologist, and even scrub in on a surgery. I discuss cases with other infectious diseases specialists if I cannot give a satisfactory answer after seeing the patient. These experiences refine the information and can sometimes permit a physician to detect things that went unnoticed before.

Sometimes a referral to a specialist can be helpful to review the case again and move past any bias. Sometimes a person may have a syndrome that a specialist's system 1 (intuitive) decision-making can detect. I once diagnosed a patient with atrial fibrillation in the ID clinic after an unexpected exam finding of an uneven pulse. The patient thought he had a tick-borne disease that was causing him to feel breathless. After seeing his provider and being told that it was unlikely, he insisted on getting a referral to infectious diseases. I found it satisfying and humorous to order an ECG after the visit.

Tips for Approaching Challenging Diagnoses

1. Go Back to the History and Exam
2. Keep Open Communication
3. Go Toward the Place of Greatest Change
4. Watchful Waiting with Diligent Follow-up
5. Consider Collaboration and a Second Opinion

Final Thoughts on Difficult Cases: Technology May Provide More Certainty

Is there a role for other diagnostic options or to treat early in challenging cases? It all depends on the level of acuity and the risk of waiting. Sometimes, a physician can treat patients while closely watching them and considering other causes. However, it is always preferable to wait for treatment until after a definitive diagnosis is made. I have seen infectious disease doctors try "steroid challenges" on febrile patients that they did not think had infections. Occasionally what one believes to be an inflammatory process may end up being an infection "on steroids." Infectious diseases worsen on steroids, including common bacterial infections, fungal infections, and miliary tuberculosis.[41]

Technology might equip doctors with the capabilities of diagnosing challenging infectious diseases earlier. New tests, such as the whole genome next-generation sequencing, may be game-changers with the potential to detect 1,000 different microbial pathogens from a sample of blood or a "blood biopsy" (Gu et al., 2019). These tests have high sensitivity (75%) and specificity (92%) in sepsis patients, even after negative blood cultures (Lecuit, 2014). They are not yet widely available and cost-effective for routine use[42]. However, as the technology improves and other companies offer their options, the prices will likely drop. It may redefine how doctors practice medicine. Imagine any patient acutely ill in the emergency department getting a blood test that could identify an infectious etiology within hours.

Cancer screening is going in the direction of being less invasive. Traditionally, screening for colorectal cancer has required a colonoscopy. Many stool- and blood-based studies are now available for detecting certain cancers earlier. These tests look for colon cancer biomarkers and are not only less invasive but have high specificity (92% for blood-based) (Ladabaum, 2013). However, the blood-based test has low sensitivity (48%) compared to the fecal immunochemical tests (FIT) (73-92%), meaning that, if used alone, it could miss more than half of colon cancers (Ebner, 2020).

In summary, there are times in a physician's practice when there is discomfort in making a diagnosis—sometimes, the pieces do not add up. It forces a physician to consider alternative causes and reframe prior interpretations. It is crucial to embrace these situations and remember that a patient is wrestling with this uncertainty. Strong doctor-patient and doctor-doctor collaborations are vital to push ahead.

Sudden Health Changes

One of the most challenging experiences is witnessing a sudden change in someone's health. Doctors listen to patients explain the stories of how their lives went from a steady state to one of change and turbulence. Whatever patients are grappling with, physicians aspire to meet it with open ears and offer advice in approaching the workup. Physicians are truly blessed and privileged with an opportunity to be a guide and confidant to others on their health journey—and ultimately, their life journey.

In most cases, a physician formulates a plan for a developing condition over several visits. However, sometimes the changes can occur like a lightning strike. Rapid changes shift the pace and priority of workup and treatment, forcing physicians to make more impactful decisions faster or witness something they may not have the resources to correct.

According to the American Heart Association, 475,000 Americans die yearly from cardiac arrest. The likelihood of surviving a cardiac arrest is only 10 percent outside of the hospital.

It does improve with cardiopulmonary resuscitation (CPR) but not as much as in the hospital. One study showed in-hospital CPR for cardiopulmonary arrest had a 30.4 percent success rate; only 12 percent were alive at discharge (Saghafania, 2010). A student or resident begins to address these emergencies with advanced cardiac life support (ACLS) training. After running a few codes in the hospital, they realize it is not likely that someone will survive—much less likely they will make it to discharge.

Conditions with the most significant risk involve the body's most critical systems (**Table 3**). Many of them are infectious, cardiovascular, and neurologic insults. They often result when a more extensive process causes instability not relieved through the body's homeostatic mechanisms. However, any considerable perturbation or trauma can become life-threatening when it rapidly impacts the airways, leads to acute blood loss, injures the brain, or taxes the heart. For example, a patient may have abdominal pain from a peptic ulcer for months, but only after it erodes into the stomach's larger vascular supply does hemorrhage result, and significant blood loss occurs rapidly.

Although the body can adapt to changes if disease develops slowly, rapid changes can quickly destabilize the body. Whatever may have been the original cause, a condition known as **shock** ensues from decreased blood flow and reduced oxygen delivery to the tissues. The clock starts ticking for physicians to determine the source of shock, correct it, if possible, and provide supportive care.

Case 14: "Doctor, I Thought I Saw Blood"

As a resident, I saw a patient visiting from Germany on my emergency medicine rotation. He was a teacher, and his visit to Washington, DC was a short one, having organized a tour of the United States for his students. While walking around and touring points of interest,

Table 3: Examples of Life-threatening Conditions by System	
Neurologic: Acute cerebrovascular accident Acute bacterial meningitis Acute aneurysmal bleed Acute viral encephalitis **Cardiovascular:** Ruptured aortic aneurysm: thoracic and abdominal Ventricular fibrillation Acute bacterial endocarditis with septal perforation Acute myocardial infarction Acute pulmonary embolism Acute congestive heart failure with pulmonary edema **Respiratory:** Tension pneumothorax Acute respiratory distress syndrome Pulmonary hemorrhage (traumatic, aneurysm, etc.) **Gastrointestinal:** Ruptured viscus: gastric, duodenal, small bowel, colon Acute GI bleed: variceal bleed, peptic ulcer, diverticular.	**Genitourinary:** Fournier's gangrene Acute obstructive urinary tract infection **Gynecologic:** Amniotic fluid embolism Uterine hemorrhage from retained products of conception Eclampsia **Musculoskeletal:** Necrotizing fasciitis Compound fracture with fat embolism **Infection:** Malaria Septic Shock, multiple causes Dengue Hemorrhagic Fever Multiple Hemorrhagic viruses. **Endocrine:** Hypoglycemic coma Adrenal crisis Myxedema coma **Allergy:** Anaphylactic shock from medications, allergen, etc.

including the Washington Monument and Jefferson memorial, he developed stomach pain and nausea and had a vomiting episode. He informed me that he thought he saw blood in the vomitus. As I listened to his story, I became concerned about a bleeding peptic ulcer because he mentioned some stomach pains leading up to this.

Following our discussion, I went to the ER order board and requested that a nurse place a nasogastric tube to lavage for blood and then began seeing other patients. I reviewed the case with the ER attending. Later, after checking back on the board, I noticed that nurse was erasing my order. The attending told me that he spoke with the patient and felt that it would not likely be helpful if we pursued it further. I pressed him on it, but he had already decided not to do it. The nurse released the patient to return to his group. He felt better, and all the bloodwork was normal.

I reported for my next ER shift two days later. The German patient had returned earlier that evening. This time there was no controversy; it was undoubtedly from a gastrointestinal (GI) bleed. The ER nurse placed a nasogastric tube, and a saline lavage revealed blood. It was time to admit him to the hospital and arrange an EGD[43].

The diagnosis was not apparent until the patient had a significant bleed later and required intervention. Up until then, another possible diagnosis would be Mallory-Weiss tears, a common cause of blood seen in the vomitus[44]. These usually heal on their own and do not lead to severe bleeding. Given the normal bloodwork, the attending decided that the patient could monitor himself and come back if needed for future bleeding.

Disagreements often come up with patient management between attending and trainee. They offer an opportunity to find ways to collaborate and further clarify plans. It is always helpful to go back to the patient's account. If the attending and resident saw the patient together, it may have led to a more unified front in the decision-making process since the patient could have voiced his observations and concerns to both parties.

Case 15: The Last Bleed

The twelve-bed Intensive Care Unit (ICU) at the veteran's hospital where I trained was a crowded, busy place with many physician teams coming and going. I was a first-year resident, and it was my month for an intensive experience. A patient with cirrhosis came in for confusion[45] secondary to liver disease from Hepatitis C. He had bleeding from esophageal varices. These are swollen veins lining the esophagus that occur after veins back up from a scarred liver.

A GI doctor performed an endoscopy on the patient and injected epinephrine into the varices to tighten the vessel and hopefully stop the bleeding. He still had a trickle of blood loss, evidenced by the steady drop in his red blood cell markers. The intensivist decided to observe him for another few days in the ICU to ensure that the bleeding stopped. He could receive blood products and fluids more easily there if he needed them.

The morning of the event was unremarkable. The interns and residents reported for rounds with the intensivist, a bright, exemplary physician. While rounding, the nurse caring for the cirrhotic patient informed us that he had a vomiting episode showing scant blood. We took note of that and continued rounding. We planned to address it when we had time to talk with him.

The nurse alerted us again. It looked like it could not wait. He had respiratory concerns, and his blood pressure was dropping. The attending stopped the rounds and went to his bedside. The patient's pressure was falling, and as he drifted into unconsciousness, he now had a threatened airway. The nurse placed the head of the bed down in the Trendelenburg position; the maneuver improves blood flow to the brain in someone with shock.

When a person shows signs or impending risk of respiratory arrest, a doctor inserts a tube into the mouth, through the epiglottis, and into the trachea. The tube connects to a ventilator that provides life-saving oxygen and ventilation. The intern on the case was a sharp, tenacious emergency medicine resident. She rushed to the head of the bed, preparing to intubate him.

While she readied herself for the procedure, the patient suddenly vomited again. This time it was bright red blood and not a tiny amount. It was a full-on hemorrhage. We watched as the patient bled out in front of us. She tried to intubate him; bright red, infectious blood splashed on her face and goggles. Blood filled his mouth as she tried to visualize where to insert the tube. Attempts to resuscitate him failed. No blood products could arrive as quickly as he needed them. It was his last bleed, and we could do nothing for him.

It was devastating for me to see a person die this way in front of my eyes. It took me some time to process his death and avoid more accessible coping methods (e.g., alcohol). At that stage in my training, it was not the first time, nor would it be the last, that I would have to witness a patient's transition from life to death.

Case 16: A Stroke of Misfortune

I saw a hospitalized patient for an infectious disease consultation. She had bacteria growing in her blood. She was in her late seventies and noticed a decline in her usual state of health over two to three weeks. During that time, she grew weaker and more tired. There were no accompanying fevers, but she did have an episode of rigors, shaking chills, one week before her admission. She went to the emergency department for increasing fatigue. The ER workup identified low blood pressure and a high white blood cell count.

The lab contacted the physician, alerting him that her blood cultures became positive for *Aeromonas*, an uncommon bacteria. A doctor orders a new set after a person has positive blood cultures. The hospitalist decided to discharge her on oral antibiotics so long as she had a prompt follow-up to ensure the cultures remained negative. She felt better and agreed. The source of the organism was still unclear.

When a patient has persistently positive blood cultures, that is a tell-tale sign of an infection within the vascular system, most commonly one of the heart valves— a condition known as endocarditis. While *Aeromonas* is not a common cause of bloodstream infections, any bacteria can cause endocarditis. She had a trans-thoracic echocardiogram (TTE), a specialized chest ultrasound that assesses heart function and looks for signs of infectious growth on a valve known as *vegetation*. Her original ECHO did not show any apparent vegetation and only mild mitral valve issues.

I saw her after a more sensitive test, the trans-esophageal Echo (TEE), showed a sudden worsening in her valve function and confirmed the infectious growth on the valve. Her weakness progressed, and she returned to the hospital four days later. The second ECHO showed a significant mitral valve vegetation measuring greater than two centimeters. The findings materialized in only four days.

The cardiac surgeons reviewed her case with the cardiologist and believed she had no impending risk to warrant emergency valve surgery. They would consider it at a later time. Nurses started her on intravenous antibiotics. I evaluated her, asked her about her illness history, and discussed the timing of any intervention. She did not feel well but was in some way relieved to be back in the hospital to find answers. I left her bedside to return to the doctor's work room next door to begin the review of her chart and my dictation.

Approximately one hour later, I heard a "code stroke" called. My mind immediately went to the patient. When a person has a significant vegetation on the mitral or aortic valve (on the left side of the heart), there is a risk of stroke, as little pieces break off the valve into the arterial circulation and transit to any part of the body, including the brain.

The American Stroke Association uses the acronym **F.A.S.T.** to spot a stroke. The patient's nurse found her with a sudden neurologic change: a left facial droop (F), right arm paralysis (A), and speech difficulties (S). The T stands for *time*, and after witnessing her stroke, the team escorted her promptly to the radiology department for a CT scan.

An early CT scan is not entirely accurate in detecting a stroke. Still, it is a quick and valuable method to rule out a stroke associated with an inter-cerebral bleed (hemorrhagic stroke). It is not as sensitive a study for an ischemic stroke caused by an embolism (a clot) or a vegetation fragment that dislodges from the valve and enters the brain's circulation. Therefore, a normal study does not rule out an ischemic stroke. However, her CT scan was already showing changes.

When her findings suggested an acute stroke, likely from an infected heart valve, it was time to evaluate her for treatment with a *thrombectomy* or *thrombolytics*. These are two intervention options in the setting of an acute thrombotic (clot-related) stroke. A thrombectomy is when doctors introduce a small, specialized probe into circulation to remove the clot. Thrombolytics are medications that break up clots that impede circulation. Interventionalists[46] administer the therapy intravenously or directly into the cerebral vascular system (El Tawil, 2017).

When I saw her, I quickly determined that she had a stroke from the above changes. I spoke to her gently, "You had a stroke. We will get you evaluated promptly and address this with the options available. You are going to be OK." The statement did not expose my fears of her poor prognosis. As it occurred in a split second, I wanted to give her support rather than a report on the outlook.

She acknowledged my comment. She reached out with her functioning arm, and I held her hand for a moment, ignoring the warnings about shaking hands during a pandemic. *If there were ever a time to hold someone's hand, it would be now*, I thought. Like the flick of a light switch, she faced these sudden changes in her body, alone in her head, unable to express her feelings.

The doctors referred her to another center to have an urgent intervention. "Time is brain." After an ischemic stroke, studies show that the brain loses approximately two million neurons per minute in the affected area (Saver, 2006). Unfortunately, the intervention was unsuccessful in returning the flow to the affected cerebral artery. The neuro-interventionalists posited that the blockage was from valve tissue that had broken off and traversed up to the left middle cerebral artery. There was no reversing this process.

In the United States, a stroke ranks as the fifth leading cause of death. For survivors, a return of function occurs over ensuing days to even as late as six months. Although recovery depends on the severity of the stroke and underlying conditions, only 10 percent of people experience a full recovery after a stroke. The rest fall into three categories: 25 percent continue to suffer minor problems, 40 percent are moderate to severely impaired, and 10 percent require long-term care (ASA).

A significant stroke attacks a person's steady-state and alters them forever. Someone who survives faces an uphill course of adjusting to a drastic change. The only recourse is to adapt, modify, and rebuild. Although this patient's stroke resulted from infection, most strokes are related to a chronic health condition, like diabetes or hypertension. It motivates me as a physician to target prevention to reduce the risk of stroke and its toll on individuals and their families.

Case 17: When a Visitor Becomes a Patient

It was another busy morning on infectious diseases rounds during my work as an attending. I returned to the Intensive Care Unit to check on a patient. I walked through the unit's hallway and noticed a woman in her early fifties coming toward me. She looked dizzy and pale, leaning toward the wall as though she were about to fall. She was not responding to me, so I helped her safely down to the floor.

The adrenaline rushed through me as I began to assess her. She was unresponsive, so I told the nurse to call a *code blue*, an alarm to get physicians, nurses, and respiratory therapists to the scene. It takes teamwork for the best attempts to save a life with cardiopulmonary resuscitation. Meanwhile, I asked for an automated external defibrillator (AED) and began CPR on the floor.

We got her on a stretcher and wheeled her into a room in the intensive care unit while continuing the code. A few more nurses joined in, and we took turns administering CPR, counting out thirty beats followed by a brief pause to provide respirations. I applied the automated defibrillator; it did not detect a shockable rhythm. As I read the monitor, it showed a flatline meaning no electrical or mechanical activity of the heart. *Damn, this is asystole*, I thought, as my own heart seemed to stop for a moment. Asystole portends a dismal prognosis[47]. After about twenty minutes, we called off the CPR and terminated efforts. The visitor who instantly became a patient had the briefest hospitalization.

Although it was not completely clear what happened, it was conceivable that she developed a blood clot (DVT[48]) in her peripheral circulation. She had traveled and at least satisfied one of the tenets of *Virchow's triad*: stasis; the others are hypercoagulable state and vessel wall injury. A clot in a leg vein may have moved through the circulation to the right side of the heart and then gotten pumped into the lung's circulation. The condition is known as a pulmonary embolism (PE), and it can kill. The CDC estimates that one in four people who have a PE will die— approximately one hundred thousand people yearly.

I thought about how devastating it would be for her family to hear the news: the wicked irony of a woman who was not even a patient lying dead in the same intensive care unit where her sister was fighting for her life.

Managing Grief in Medicine

Death is a part of life. The care of patients comes with the possibility that they will not survive. Becoming a doctor requires being in touch with our vulnerabilities and relationship with death.

As a nocturnist (moonlighter) during my fellowship, the nurses frequently called me to check on unstable patients. Despite all our best efforts, some of these patients did not survive the shift. Later the nurse would call me to pronounce an individual dead. I would walk into the room and imagine a soul exiting their now lifeless body. I took my job solemnly as I examined the body: a sternal rub confirmed unresponsiveness; there was no chest movement, pupillary reaction, or heart sounds.

Just as I held a patient's hand in prayer as they lay dying, I did the same to a dead body— a symbolic gesture to reflect on the sanctity of life. I would then telephone the family and inform them of their loved one's passing. Sometimes the family questioned the declaration as if holding on and not accepting their loved one's death. The reactions ranged from anger to acceptance. I held space with them, listening to their responses and offering words of support. The more I addressed death peacefully and openly, the more perspective it gave me to be present compassionately. A person's death reminds us of our own mortality and is a call to action.

Even as I took a vacation traveling through Ecuador as an intern, I confronted my relationship with death head-on. After a four-day Amazon tour, our vehicle passed a group of people huddled on the side of the road. The mountain pass was narrow and overlooked a cliff. I asked the driver to stop, opened the door, and a woman cradling a small girl came forward, crying and shouting to get our attention. A large truck struck her daughter, and she was unresponsive.

I signaled her to come inside the car, and we drove to the only hospital in Baños. Two doctors awaited as I carried the girl in, and we conducted an examination together. She had a blown right pupil and a large bruise on her abdomen, signifying intracranial and intraabdominal bleeding. The doctors responded flatly that there were no neurosurgery services and that she would not survive the trip to Quito. There was nothing else anyone could offer, and I imagined that her options were minimal, even if we were in the United States. It was a saddening experience for me as I observed the mother's reaction after the doctors coldly told her of her daughter's prognosis.

To see a life lost before one's eyes is a poignant lesson on the limitations of medicine. These events continue to challenge me to understand my role as a physician and look for ways to promote health and prevent untimely death. Although everyone's life eventually must end, death leaves a stain on a physician's heart and psyche that requires processing. A physician often responds to a patient's death with the grief of losing someone and a sense of personal responsibility. Nevertheless, we can enhance the way we cope by self-care measures, understanding life's interconnectedness with death— moving past the initial feelings of guilt or blame, and creating a supportive environment to discuss grief (Shute, 2019).

We must refrain from simply forgetting (amnesia) or numbing ourselves (anesthesia) from a loss (Weller, 2015). Psychotherapist Francis Weller refers to these approaches to grief as the "primary sins of Western civilization" (Weller, 2015). It is easier than ever to escape the pain of the memory by keeping busy, filling in the empty spaces of time with technology, substance use, and other distractions. However, one needs to directly face their fears and pain to process grief and heal stronger as a result.

Embrace your grief, for there your soul will grow.
—Carl Jung

CHAPTER 7

The Difficult Encounter

Key Points

• Not all encounters are productive; there may be malignant motives. A physician who clarifies care objectives and sets boundaries can ensure a favorable outcome.

• Opiate dependence resulted in the untimely death of more than 760,000 people from 1999 to 2018.

• Seventy to ninety percent of communication is nonverbal. A doctor may develop a skillset to detect untruths through body language.

Cases

Case 18: New in Town

Case 19: Going with the Momentum

The Doctor-Patient Relationship and Understanding Motives

A clinic serves as a meeting place for patients to express their concerns and get answers in the form of a thorough evaluation, additional workup, and therapy. A therapeutic physician-patient relationship relies on mutual trust. Both parties benefit from accuracy, honesty, and confidentiality as they share information.

I make a great effort to listen to patients' comments and observe body language as they explain their concerns. Within a patient's words lie the clues to the motives for seeking care, mitigating pain or illness, or allaying an underlying fear. The physician gains rapport when they can pinpoint the concerns and acknowledge the person speaking the words. Patients can express their motives clearly or keep them buried in words— both said and not said. Intentions may be sincere, or they can be disingenuous or malingering.[49]

Doctors are generally not comfortable doubting or distrusting a patient's words. In some patient interactions, alarms may sound in the communication style and comments that suggest an ulterior motive. While this chapter only briefly reviews the opiate epidemic, the role of opiate medications in chronic pain remains controversial. Specific patients benefit from opiates under close physician observation. However, there is no doubt that increasing pain medication prescriptions can fuel more frequent encounters by individuals with aberrant behaviors[50] and ulterior motives.

Barriers, Motives, and Hidden Agendas

Patient communication barriers often develop after negative experiences with doctors in the past. Some patients report callous statements from their doctors. Sometimes a little courage and compassion are needed to tackle medical concerns, especially if they are tied to maladaptive behaviors. Usually, a brief exchange that acknowledges the person behind the complaint is often the most crucial step to building rapport and bridging the two parties.

Patients seeking care and finding answers usually have nothing to hide; their intentions lie in understanding and narrowing in on the potential cause of their concerns. Each word brings a physician and patient closer to clarity and agreement on the direction of the work-up. However, there are some exceptions to accepting the validity of a patient's story, particularly when it comes to pain medications and other controlled substances. Anything that calls to question one aspect of the history disrupts the legitimacy of the entire visit.

When a patient deliberately conceals details, for example, someone with ulterior motives, it can undermine any attempts to help. Their true intention is not for collaboration or assistance—it is for manipulation and deceit. Early on, I observed that some people were willing to risk getting kicked out of the clinic for the possibility of scoring pain medications. Their objective was never to develop a doctor-patient relationship.

I admit that I wrestled with "trust but verify" because it initially stifles a developing partnership. However, most people without ulterior motives understand the reason for the questions. I learned the hard way not to immediately trust every patient[51], listening for warning signs in their answers or my "gut feeling." I would take the time to review their records and confirm the details. Often, a few more visits brought reassurance and clarity of the patient's intentions, including dishonesty.

Through experience, I developed a sensitized ear to listen for potential clues to opiate use disorder, to review in detail each medication, their indications, and the reasons for changing physicians. Many patients seeking new opiate prescriptions never informed their prior physician that they were changing doctors. It can be an excellent time to connect with the previous doctor in preparing clinic visit notes. I was often surprised by how valuable a phone call was to clarify a patient's motives.

With the United States' disjointed healthcare system, changing physicians or "doctor shopping[52]" while concealing the recent visit information is possible. A mandated system reduces overall controlled substance prescribing and the amount of risky and redundant prescriptions (Strickler, 2019). The Prescription and Drug Monitoring Program (PDMP) provides a way to track prior controlled substance prescriptions and ordering physicians.

However, the programs do not always allow access to the out-of-state activity. For this reason, someone requesting controlled substance prescriptions on the first visit, having relocated from out-of-state and not furnishing prior physician information, is a considerable risk of gaming the system. Often there are inconsistencies, subtle and not so subtle, that suggest ulterior motives.

Deception in the Clinic

How does a person respond when they hear misinformation or an untruth? They naturally process the information, weigh the likelihoods, and look for motivations. The intention often lies within the potential reasons for the request, the chosen words, and the nonverbal cues of the messenger. Many telling phrases reveal a potentially problematic doctor-patient relationship[53]. "I stopped seeing that doctor because he flat-out told me that he wouldn't increase my medications;" "We disagreed with the number of pain medications I should receive;" "That clinic didn't care about my pain, but you and your staff seem like you care."

If this exercise suggests dishonesty or manipulation, one can discover a potential motive through follow-up questions, setting judgment aside. When reduced to a common denominator, lies come from a conscious and subconscious attempt to conceal behavior. It may be that a patient is not ready to reveal what they might construe as harmful or shameful if known. A lie attempts to distort an event's facts that correspond to a genuine motive. A person perceives a lie as less painful or more beneficial than exposing the truth, usually because it may be regarded as a negative, unexpected, harmful, or outright illegal behavior.

Body Language and Detecting Untruths

The body communicates with more than words. As much as 70 to 90 percent of communication occurs nonverbally, even as words come out. If a person fabricates a story, they require a significant level of concentration to stay consistent. Simultaneously, the brain responds to the stress, releasing hormones cortisol, epinephrine, and norepinephrine. Invariably the body forecasts changes: pupils dilate, respiratory rate increases, the mouth becomes dry, blinking increases, and the person rubs and scratches the nose and ears. Body movements can reveal a liar, such as a change from their baseline mannerisms as they tell a lie. Changes include shaking a limb, moving back and forth, tilting their head, or leaning toward the door (Palmieri, 2009).

I saw a patient found on bloodwork to have a sexually transmitted infection (STI) and asked how he thought he acquired it. His response was, "I don't know." As I pressed further, explaining how the disease could be transmitted, I noticed his posture change. He repeatedly sat forward and began to move his left leg, and his voice cracked as he answered. Although I had asked his wife to step out briefly, he did not want to discuss it further—perhaps to keep it out of the chart.

As he responded, I asked myself some questions. Was he still reconciling the guilt of infidelity? Was he avoiding rebuke or worse if his wife knew? She had acquired the same disease. *She's likely already figured it out by now*, I thought. I came upon a brick wall. Rather than push through it, I decided that I could still treat him for the condition, without knowing the details, if he knew how to protect himself from future STIs .

Every person develops a different skill to determine untruths. I was very gullible as a child, accepting every statement as truth. After all, I followed an honesty principle. I expected the same from everyone. Sometimes, that got me into trouble believing lies, sarcasm, or jokes. I developed better detective skills as a doctor and then as a parent. Is it not true that most parents can tell when their children are dishonest? The child's intention may be to continue something otherwise restricted or curtailed by the parents (e.g., snacks, video games, staying up late). The story is often contrived and illogical. It may evolve and show more inconsistencies as the parent asks the child to explain further. They might use words or phrases in an attempt to disperse focus from them. Maintaining consistency in a lie is mentally challenging and taxing on the body. Just ask a person who is lying to repeat their story backward.

Often a feeling of shame or embarrassment may hold a person to an untruth. It is one of the greatest privileges of a doctor to be a resource to a patient when they can finally face this shame and vocalize their feelings with their doctor as a witness. The release of guilt is often the most crucial step in processing and reconciling feelings, discussing them with other loved ones, and moving toward a behavior change.

The cases in this chapter are about another category of deception: seeking to manipulate the health system for one's gain while others pay the price. First, I start with an overview of the opiate epidemic.

Addiction and the Opiate Epidemic[54]

The opioid crisis in the US has led to more than 760,000 people dying from overdoses between 1999 and 2018 (USDHHS). Each day, an estimated 130 people die from opioid-related causes. The pharmaceutical industry launched a decade-long strategy to sell various formulations of opiates to manage pain. Pain medications, or opiates, became increasingly prescribed in the late eighties and nineties when reports suggested improvements in quality of life through their use for those suffering from chronic noncancer pain (Portenoy 1986). Pain became the fifth vital sign,[55] incorporating a pain scale to make a subjective experience more objective. Addressing pain was considered a patient satisfaction marker.

While the pharmaceutical companies' pockets deepened, liberal prescribing of opiates for pain resulted in more harm than benefit. Yet, there was no change in the amount of pain reported on patient surveys (Chang, 2014). The opiate crisis hit rural areas particularly hard. In some states, such as West Virginia, Kentucky, and South Carolina, pain pills were high enough to amount to every person getting 66.5, 63.3, and 58 pills per year, respectively. In 2018, more than 67,300 Americans died from drug-involved overdoses, both from illicit drugs and prescription opiates (NIDA).

Pain medications such as oxycodone, hydrocodone, and morphine, create dependence and, in a way, lead to more pain. Opiates act on the brain's pain area, or nociceptive pathway, where the medications promote changes in the brain. They attach to opioid receptors on neurons, known as *mu receptors*, triggering the release of neurotransmitters, such as dopamine, which activate the rewards pathway (mesolimbic reward system) and create a sensation of pleasure and decreased pain. Over time, the receptors become downregulated and less responsive to the dose, requiring a more significant amount for a similar effect; this blunting effect is known as *tolerance*.

At the same time, opiates decrease the production of noradrenaline (NA)[56] in the *locus ceruleus* (LC), a concentrated production area of this neurotransmitter. It contributes to bodily responses, including blood pressure, breathing, and alertness. Opiate use leads to a compensatory increased production of NA, which competes with the effect of the opiate, and in the setting of a disruption of opiate use, contributes to the signs of opiate withdrawal (Kosten, 2002).

As a result of pleasure from opiates, the brain biologically alters to maintain the behavior. A new pain results: the pain of withdrawal. The displeasure from opiate withdrawal may be enough to provoke cravings and opiate reuse. Addictive behaviors develop, including preoccupation with these medications, dose-escalation, and drug-seeking behavior (Evans, 2016).

With the opiate crackdown in the last few years, many people faced drug dependence, while doctors quickly tapered patients off their longstanding medications. Meanwhile, opiates were also indirectly used to medicate underlying anxiety and depression. Patients receiving chronic pain medications commonly had co-associated depression, with some studies showing a prevalence of up to 60 percent, half of these in a more severe category (Rayner, 2016). Sadly, with the reduction of prescriptions in the last several years, those unsuccessful at opiate cessation found comparable drugs on the illegal market, including heroin.

Over 12 months ending in April 2021, while the nation grappled with the COVID-19 pandemic, there were more than 100 thousand drug overdose deaths, an almost 30% increase from the year before (CDC 2021). Not all these deaths were due to street drugs. The CDC estimates that over 28% of all opioid deaths (2019) were from prescription opioids like fentanyl and methadone (CDC).

Doctors continue to be at the front line of the opioid epidemic with increasing fallout. An estimated 11% to 40% of US adults live with chronic pain (IPRCC, 2016). In primary care, about 1 in 4 patients prescribed opioids takes them differently than the instructions, and 1 in 10 show signs of opioid use disorder (Sokol, 2021). In keeping with the biopsychosocial model, pain is more than a dysfunction that needs a prescription. Pain manifests both as a physical signal and the brain's recognition of it (Gatchel, 2007). A multidisciplinary approach offers therapeutic modalities that can reduce pain, improve mobility, and decrease the need for medications.

Case 18: New in Town

A person may use their history, including medical conditions, as a rationale or justification for maintaining a behavior. A thirty-year-old man made an appointment with me for a new patient visit. He had just moved to Oregon and requested a new pain medication prescription. After a motor vehicle accident, he had two back surgeries, and the second one involved the placement of stabilization rods.

We talked about his past medications. He took three to four hydrocodone (Vicodin) tablets daily for chronic back pain before his move. At the visit, he had been out of them for several weeks. Although he had effectively gone through withdrawal after his last prescription ran out, he was interested in starting them again. He provided no further details about who managed his medications other than his interest in resuming the same dose.

I asked the patient if he expected me to write a new prescription after an initial visit. He may have sensed a degree of reservation in my voice. He proceeded to tell me with a smile that, although he could do without it, he does much better with it. The candid statement suggested a motive behind the visit. I thought he might be concealing a craving to resume opiate use, not to treat pain. I kindly declined, raised my concern about the behavior, and asked him to check back with me for a follow-up. He never returned.

Case 19: Going with the Momentum

The body sends signals to the brain telling us of a site of inflammation or dysfunction. One of the cardinal signs of inflammation is *dolor*[57] or pain. Pain is a vital sensation that alerts us of potential harm. It can be challenging to determine when someone taking pain medications may need closer evaluation. Sometimes acute worsening of pain can be misattributed to a person's chronic pain issues. It might seem sensible to escalate the dose of pain medications for increased back pain, only to discover it came from a kidney stone or a complicated urinary tract infection. Consequently, medicines that blunt the pain signals can mask serious issues, including diseases requiring surgical attention.

The emergency department is the most common location for addressing acute pain. Before the current limitations on the number of pain medication tablets prescribed in the ER setting, the emergency department was an access point for opiate dependence. Chronic dependence on opiates leads to a preoccupation with these medications and drug-seeking behavior. Occasionally, someone who is malingering[58] may present to the ER with pain, go undetected, and receive treatment.

A patient came into the ER for increasing back pain. He had a prior lower back (lumbar spine) surgery several years before but reported a recent worsening of pain. The attending physician examined him and ordered lumbar spine X-rays. After ruling out any underlying conditions, the physician prescribed a five-day course of pain medications. He appointed the patient to the on-call primary care doctor (me) for a new patient visit.

I met the patient on his ER follow-up visit, took a basic history, and performed an exam. He had a midline scar from his prior surgery and grimaced as I touched his back and moved his legs. The findings suggested musculo-ligamentous back pain (lumbago) with no warning signs of disc disease. He was in my clinic and out of hydrocodone. He stated that they were helping and that he did not find any benefit in nonsteroidal medications, like ibuprofen or naproxen.

It was the first time I had met him, and I was not able to verify much from the records. I could not conclude he had an acute flare-up other than a stiff back. I decided to provide him with an additional short course of pain medications and a physical therapy referral. He followed up again in another week.

I remember reviewing his social history. He did not smoke or drink alcohol. Given that weeks of pain could impact his ability to work, I asked him about his occupation. He stated that he "sold things on the internet." I wondered why he gave such a cryptic response, even after asking him to explain further. I scheduled him for another short visit in one week and gave him another prescription for the pain medications.

He returned with persistent pain. He did not make an appointment with physical therapy, claiming he would make one after the day's visit. I had him come in for three visits to monitor his behavior. Each time he came into the clinic, he did not elaborate on his symptoms. He stated that his back pain continued and that the pain medications helped a little. His back pain concerns weren't fitting the expected duration of an acute exacerbation. He was not taking self-care initiatives such as stretching or following through with a referral to physical therapy.

It seemed like he was concealing his motives. His words said one thing, but his body and comments told me something else. After I questioned the need for ongoing pain medications for acute back pain, I told him that I would need to check a urine tox screen. He immediately changed his body posture, slumping back in his chair, and responded flatly, "I'm going to need a glass of water to go."

Three days later, I called him to tell him that we could no longer prescribe pain medications because the urine tox result showed he violated the pain contract. The urine toxicology screen was positive for benzodiazepines, muscle relaxants, hydromorphone (Dilaudid), and marijuana. However, the urine did not show the hydrocodone I prescribed him. He immediately responded, "Are you saying I am no more than a common criminal to have those substances in my urine?" My mind went back to the comment that he "sold things on the internet," and I began to wonder if he was revealing in his question that he was indeed a criminal.

I responded, "I did not say those words. You did." He retorted in a threatening way, "What if I decide to give you a bad online rating?" I held my tongue after that statement. I suddenly realized that a phone call may not have been the best choice to discuss these findings. His words were an attempt to manipulate me. I repeated the plan to him and hung up the phone with a tense feeling. I pondered whether it was my role to alert authorities of suspicious activity but decided against it.

A few days later, I googled my name and discovered a recent anonymous review: "I won't go back to that clinic until they fire his "a--" Was that written by him?

Letting Go of Judgement and Moving On

Although it is important to be clear on setting boundaries and following guidelines in the clinic, it is often best not to confront someone directly who may be malingering. And it is not just about negative ratings. False accusations, litigation, and violence may occur as individuals attempt to defend themselves or seek retaliation. Instead, physicians should rely on the physical findings and can offer patients logical explanations, emphasizing what is within a reasonable practice (Alozai, 2021). Oftentimes, patients will move on when clear boundaries are made.

The effects of any negative interaction can linger in both patients and physicians. An individual can still offer kindness and compassion for a fellow human being. It can be challenging not to call a person out when they are actively falsifying information or feigning an illness to obtain a prescription or other benefit. We cannot begin to know the difficulties they may face to make these choices. Author Ian Maclaren's quote resonates when addressing these individuals: "Be kind, for everyone you meet is fighting a hard battle."

CHAPTER 8

On Listening, Communication, and Collaboration

Good communication is the bridge between confusion and clarity.
—Nat Turner

Great discoveries and improvements invariably involve the cooperation of many minds.
—Alexander Graham Bell

Key Points

- Active listening enables a physician and patient to connect more closely, reducing the effect of bias and allowing a closer perspective to a patient's concerns.
- Physician collaboration enhances patient care, harnessing the experience and skillsets of multiple physicians toward the cause

Cases

Case 20: "Oh, By the Way, Doctor…"

Case 21: A Surgeon, an ID Doc, and the Patient in the Middle

Case 22: When a UTI is not a UTI

In the Zulu language of South Africa, there is a standard greeting that goes like this: the caller states *Sikhona*, meaning "I am here to be seen," and the receiver responds *Sawubona*, meaning "I see you." The English word "respect" comes from the Latin *respicere* or to "look back at" — another reference to sight (Murphy-Shigematsu, 2021). As we acknowledge someone's presence, we *see* them as fellow humans and create a space for respect and communication. In preparing to become a doctor, students benefit by learning how to harness the power of words and the skill of listening. Effective communication allows one a pathway to understanding another's concerns, but it also recognizes the hopes and fears that contribute to them. Effectively, the listener sees the humanity of the person behind the words.

Recall the nine core competencies associated with medical school success in chapter 1. Several of them fit into the communication skillset: social skills, oral communication, cultural competence, and teamwork (Koenig T, 2013). These abilities are not taught as easily as the basic sciences are. Often, they must be fashioned through dynamic instruction, feedback, and ongoing practice.

Listening: A Lost Art of Medicine?

Listening is as much a science as an art form. It creates a bridge between sender and receiver. Rather than simply hearing words, listening requires development, patience, and attention. Indeed, it is one of the essential tools in a physician's toolbox . In the clinic, both doctors and patients benefit from prioritizing communication. Sir William Osler's declaration to "listen to the patient long enough, and they will tell you what's wrong with them" is true but jeopardized by the many interruptions commonly seen in today's clinics (Platt, 1974; Peterson, 1992) .

If you see a doctor today, you may notice a rift between the business of medical practice and the skill of listening. Doctors sometimes feel forced to truncate listening in the fast-paced clinic to keep up with charting and a demanding schedule. Listening is becoming a lost art, and its absence compromises patient care. Although helpful to recap information, a short, focused interview often closes the door to understanding early on. The average time a patient gets to speak before being interrupted is 12 seconds. (Rhoades, 2001). In another observational study, resident physicians interrupted patients twice on average during a total time of four minutes. Female patients were interrupted more often, and female residents interrupted patients less (Rhoades, 2001).

Aside from the interruptions and shorter time for a patient to speak, there are myriad distractions in the clinic, including a barrage of door knocks, phone calls, and text message alerts. Electronic Medical Records (EMR) may have begun with the prospect of organizing and enhancing access to medical records, but it can stifle the flow during the information-gathering stage.

The EMR is here to stay. Unfortunately, it requires extra time to complete it—even more than seeing patients. In an observational study of 982 visits, the mean length of the visit was 35.8 minutes, with 16.5 minutes face-to-face with a patient and 18.6 minutes on the EMR (Young, 2018). The physician spends about one-third of the time looking at computer screens during the visit. Doctors may miss nonverbal cues when their eyes are fixed on screens as patients communicate.

Why Listening is a Priority

A busy physician sees about four patients hourly; a regular day may amount to fifteen to twenty patient visits. It is not unusual that the visit time exceeds the scheduled time. Doctors and patients have different dynamics that are often in conflict and might impact the quality of the interview. Patients would like to ensure that they have enough time to explain their concerns and get value from the visit. The doctor factors both the patient's needs and the flow of the day. When a doctor runs behind, their ability to listen becomes even more compromised.

A physician skilled in interviewing enhances the clarity and yield of information. During the first part of the medical interview, a patient often explains their reason, or agenda , for a visit. A physician might solicit this directly if the patient did not mention it in the opening statement. In one study, only one-quarter of patients could complete their agenda without interruption (Dyche, 2005). Not determining a patient's agenda significantly impaired the physician's index of understanding (IOU) (Dyche, 2005). A reduced IOU hampers an accurate picture, leading to misdiagnoses, unnecessary tests, and incorrect treatments.

From "Difficult Patient" to Successful Visit

Not all visits go smoothly. Clinicians rated 1 in 6 visits as "difficult" in one study (Jackson, 1999). Did these encounters occur because of a "difficult patient" or other factors? Physicians were more likely to report a negative visit when patients had mood disorders and various symptoms, including more severe ones (Jackson, 1999).

However, patient complexity was not the entire story. Studies to identify the factors behind the "difficult visit" revealed that it had more to do with the physician than the patient (Mathers, 1995). These criteria included a lack of training in communication and counseling, lower job satisfaction, and a more significant workload perception. Both physicians and patients feel strained in a challenging interaction. However, when physicians develop psychosocial communication skills and ensure work-life balance, they can have a more productive, satisfying patient interaction.

Positive interaction not only improves patient care but also protects physicians from malpractice. In a look at litigated complaints in medical practice, almost one-third came from strained doctor-patient relationships and a breakdown in communication (Roter, 2006). Furthermore, there may be a discrepancy between how a doctor believed an interaction went and the patient 's conclusions. In one American Academy of Orthopedic Surgeons survey, although 75% of orthopedic surgeons felt they had communicated satisfactorily with their patients, only 21% of these patients concurred (Tong, 2005). Effective, open communication may alleviate this gap.

A beneficial interaction can increase rapport and confidence in the doctor. But what does it take to transform strained communication into effective communication? In a qualitative study of 21 vulnerable patients building a new relationship with a provider, five factors were crucial in easing anxiety and establishing trust: 1) providing reassurance, 2) inviting patients to ask questions, 3) showing patients their results and reviewing the findings, 4) avoiding language or behaviors construed as judgmental, and 5) asking patients about their treatment preferences and goals (Dang, 2017). Active listening equips a physician with the skills to address all these suggestions.

Active Listening is an Integral Part of Effective Communication

A chief complaint represents an amalgam of symptoms and signs, objective and subjective, and a patient's sensational and emotional responses. How one person uses words is as personal as how another understands them. A physician develops skills to become a professional interviewer. They wield a lexicon of key terms to categorize complaints and garner further details.

Critical to medical consultation is active listening—a communication style that is both welcoming and interactive. The ideal interview yields essential information while allowing patients to discuss their fears and concerns. Although patients may choose specific words to express their concerns, they frequently communicate another message nonverbally or emphasize subjective interpretations. When physicians actively listen, they may ask clarifying questions to fine-tune and understand the patient's agenda (Weger, 2014).

Unlike a social discussion that friends may have, a physician-patient interview aims to understand the source of a health concern. A patient's words provide clues to the problem; a physician seeks to understand the meaning and clarify the subjective gaps. Active listening creates a comfortable space for patients to express their concerns without interruption or judgment.

Time pressures and interruptions hinder the optimal flow of an effective interview. Both patient and physician may truncate communication because of these pressures, ultimately impacting the synthesis of information. Sometimes physicians can anchor on visible findings, while the exam may overlook the details of how it occurred. Communication gaps invite bias and inaccuracy. Nevertheless, physicians may understand, examine, and follow up even within a short timeframe while acknowledging the patient's concerns and appropriately directing them to a workup and treatment plan.

Strategies for Active Listening

What are some strategies for active listening to ensure an optimal interview? Though it may be challenging to avoid interruptions altogether, the office can take care in advance to limit unnecessary ones like smartphone calls, beeps, and routine patient-related questions. Staff can create a supportive environment, free of noise distraction and unencumbered by computer screens for optimal face-to-face communication.

The physician does their part to acknowledge the patient's words and show an interest in understanding. They may repeat the words a patient just used, seeking clarification. At the end of a productive visit, the doctor can inform the patient of the next steps, including lab tests or radiology, education, and the treatment pathway. If the process is not completely clear after the visit, they can discuss a timeline and follow-up strategy.

As with any other skill in medicine, a physician fine-tunes active listening through learning. Medical education should compulsorily incorporate training early on. Best communication practices need to be revisited through training, including in residency. Listening workshops for practicing physicians are also beneficial (Jagosh, 2011; Ranjan, 2015).

Table 5 includes some strategies to enhance listening. The net result is a connection that enhances a doctor's ability to objectively consider potential causes of concern, fosters a stronger doctor-patient relationship, and engenders a feeling of being understood (Weger, 2014). Excellent physician communication skills improve the quality of care, make the visit pleasant and productive, and lead to a patient's greater willingness to follow recommendations and better patient satisfaction (Stewart, 1995; Biglu, 2017) .

Table 5: Strategies of Active Listening
• Quiet, welcoming environment
• Minimize distraction
• Eye contact
• Avoid interruptions
• Visual/Verbal cue of confirmation: nodding, occasional "OK."
• Recapping: Restating the words or a summary sentence "I am hearing…" or "So you are telling me that…is that right?"
• Legitimizing concerns: "I can understand how that could lead to some concern."
• Questions from the interviewer that call for clarification or elaboration.

From Listening to Delivery

Communication was not my strong suit as a child, but it improved with practice. My medical school organized several mock-patient interviews, which allowed students to interact with patient actors on themes like eliciting the patient's agenda, delivering bad news, and addressing inappropriate statements[59]. The faculty studied our interactions for characteristics such as body language, chosen words, and delivery style. These experiences were invaluable in honing the skill.

Case 20: "Oh, and By the Way, Doctor"

I am always particularly attentive when a patient raises concern at the end of the clinic visit. There may be several reasons why a patient mentions something at the end of the visit. They may feel more comfortable by the end. The comments represent a patient's last chance to brainstorm and bring up something with the doctor. Or it is something that they have been keeping an eye on for a while and did not think it warranted a doctor's visit by itself. Patients often wait until the last minute to ask lingering questions. Whatever the reason, they are usually prefaced with, "Oh, by the way…." A physician may uncover any other concerns by asking near the end of the visit, "Anything else?" (Olson 2002).

I recall seeing an elderly patient who asked me, "Oh, by the way, what is this lump on my chest, doctor?" I had my hand on the doorknob when he asked. I turned around and agreed that it did not have to wait until the next visit. He lifted his shirt, and I placed my hand on the problem area. I detected a solid lump the size of a large walnut in the skin around his left areola—a worrisome finding that prompted a referral to the surgeon. Two weeks later, he had a mastectomy for the lump because it turned out to be breast cancer.

Collaboration in Healthcare

The World Health Organization defines collaborative practice as "multiple health workers from different professional backgrounds working together with patients, families, caregivers, and communities to deliver the highest quality of care" (WHO). A successful collaborative experience provides multiple benefits to patient care and those involved. Collaboration enhances medical decision-making, reduces the length of stay, and mitigates risks, such as morbidity and mortality, adverse drug reactions, and medication issues (Morley, 2017).

Collaboration Merges Different Perspectives

Imagine being at the scene of an accident. As you were about to cross the street, you noticed an oncoming car run through a red light, swerve into the adjacent lane, and run into another car on the side of the road you were on. You volunteered to be a witness to clarify the events. A stopped driver had an unobstructed view of the car that ran the light. However, they had a limited view when the car drove into the other lane. A pedestrian on the other side of the street had a picture of the other side of the car. When the police asked the observers and drivers to recall the events, each story was incomplete; each perspective was limited somehow. They could all agree that the car swerved out of the lane, but only the witness behind the car could confirm that the car did not run through a red light, and only the pedestrian on the opposite side of the street could verify that the car's front tire exploded and caused the car to lose control.

Each partner is a trained expert in their respective field — whether they are a therapist, nurse, hospitalist, or specialist— and provides a perspective that enhances the understanding. If only one caregiver were involved, there would be a limited scope of practice and a decreased quality of care. These patients would go without treatment that could contribute to their recovery. I am frequently reminded of this when a patient's nurse, who spends an entire shift caring for them, provides crucial input that informs medical decision-making.

D'Amour and colleagues wrote about the five concepts needed in effective collaboration: sharing, partnership, power, interdependency, and process (D'Amour, 2005). Every team member is valued, regardless of job title or training level, and relies on one another. Surrounding the patient in a home setting may be a spouse, children, siblings, or care assistant. Each person can assist with their perspective and knowledge base, often enhancing the clarity of the diagnosis, work-up, and treatment.

Healthcare benefits from a collaborative and teamwork approach. As discussed in Chapter 5, this does not necessarily mean a bunch of specialists for every disease a patient has. Collaboration requires trust and open communication, and at the center of this is the patient and their primary care provider. Whereas multiple providers could mean that each provider is "in charge" of a system or diagnosis, having a collaborative unit of providers creates an integrated partnership to discuss, evaluate, and treat as a concerted effort (Morley 2017).

Collaboration as an Infectious Diseases Specialist

As an infectious disease specialist, it is common to see patients and review the chart for underdeveloped or unclear concerns. ID doctors refer to this service as a "chart biopsy" since most of us do not perform other procedures. Sometimes, the patients have been in the hospital for days without a precise diagnosis. Collaboration becomes essential in these instances. My one visit with a patient provides only a snapshot of the entire hospitalization.

I begin by listening to the hospitalist's recollection of the patient's story, looking for areas that require clarification. Next, I review the nursing and therapy notes because these disciplines have the most frequent contact with the patient and provide insightful summaries. A chart review helps me understand the patient's baseline, the events that preceded an acute change, and the thought processes behind medical decision-making. Only after the review is complete is it time to meet the patient and discuss what is ailing them.

Details are often missing in the initial visit. After the interview, I pick up the phone and call a family member or caregiver to hear about the patient's baseline and inquire about their observations. I ask them to describe the nature of the change, whether abrupt or gradual, any associative symptoms or signs, and most importantly, what the nurse or medical assistant assessed. Frequently, the supplemental information helps address the process, e.g., the patient aspirated, choked on their food, had fallen, had additional signs or symptoms, or had their long-term foley catheter changed.

Relationships are nurtured over time and united on a common goal to improve care delivery. However, in a busy hospital setting, collaboration is far from perfect. Physicians with different rounding schedules may not be able to communicate directly with each other. Sometimes practice styles can differ: one surgeon may be more likely to explore an unresolved issue sooner, while another may observe. Or a hospitalist and ID specialist may have differing opinions on the selection of therapy. Finally, sometimes a doctor's urge to be right, which can be contagious in challenging cases, can undermine a team's goals. Ultimately, the patient's care suffers— as can that of future patients.

Case 21: A Surgeon, an ID Doc, and the Patient in the Middle

A fifty-year-old man with diabetes mellitus reported increasing pain in his right armpit (axilla.) He developed swelling that worsened over several days and fever and chills. He did not recall any pimples or other skin findings before this. He went to the emergency department, and there were clinical grounds to admit him to the hospitalist to receive intravenous antibiotics. The hospitalist consulted the surgeon and infectious diseases specialist for assistance.

A computed tomography (CT) study showed swollen tissue but no abscess or cyst. Neither did an ultrasound show a drainable collection. The initial ID specialist wondered about an abscess and recommended an incision and drainage given the size. However, after reviewing the CT scan, the surgeon decided to wait.

The patient received antibiotics while the doctors monitored him. Even after four days in the hospital, the patient's swelling only mildly improved. The surgeon recommended continuing the current IV antibiotics and monitoring. The ID specialist wrote in the chart to consider an incision and drainage. She signed out to me and informed me that the surgeon does not always receive recommendations well. She relayed that she decided to stand back and avoid confrontation with the surgeon.

As the covering specialist, I examined the patient and ran my fingers along the affected underarm. I was concerned that this was an abscess and reviewed the CT scan and ultrasound reports. I remembered the limitations of these studies for detecting developing abscesses. Studies on ultrasounds have shown high sensitivity of about 96.7 percent and lower specificity of 85.7 percent, whereas CT scans were 76 percent sensitive and 91.4 percent specific (Gaspari, 2012).

Nevertheless, sometimes the only way to be sure is to perform a needle aspirate or make an incision. The patient was open to this option. After giving a heads up to the surgeon, I numbed the area for an aspiration attempt. Despite aggressive suctioning, there was no fluid. However, I saw a scant amount of purulent fluid come out after removing the needle. The liquid was too thick to suction into the syringe.

Why not make a small stab incision, I thought, *since it's already numb?* The patient consented. There was an immediate release of pus. I contacted the surgery team to inform them of the findings, hoping they could take over. Its size and location made it a little uncomfortable for me. I figured that they could decide if the patient needed a formal incision and drainage.

I spoke with the surgeon about my findings; he seemed annoyed and hung up the phone while I was mid-sentence. I learned that day in my "green year," the first out of fellowship, what the other

ID doctors in my practice already knew: I had stepped on another physician's "turf." Maybe he construed the actions as undermining his decisions, questioning his value, or contributing to the patient's loss of faith in the surgeon. The scalpel nick had punctured deeper than just the surface of the skin.

Although my decision benefited patient care, it created a communication rift. However, the last chart notes suggested that it already existed. Afterward, the surgeon backed off and did no further procedure, writing one-sentence chart notes like, "the surgery team will continue to monitor for now." The patient's care did not suffer, but it could have. Fortunately, the swelling gradually resolved without relapse.

The surgeon and I conveniently avoided working directly together for the next few months. To me, it was not worth future toxic interactions. I also modified my practice style by only providing recommendations and avoiding procedures. After that time, the surgeon contacted me and apologized for his response to the situation. The communication brought closure to the issue, and we had smooth collaborative experiences afterward.

Case 22: When a UTI is not a UTI

An 85-year-old man with known cognitive dysfunction and chronic foley catheter came to the emergency department by ambulance from his care home. He had a change in mental status and fever. Recently, after staff noticed increased confusion and a change in color and odor of his urine, he was treated for a urinary tract infection and completed the course on the day of the new concerns[60].

In the emergency department, he was found to have an increased white blood cell count and white cells in his urine. A CT scan did not reveal any obstruction, but it did show some nonspecific signs of mild wall thickening in the colon. Nevertheless, the doctors were concerned that he still had a UTI and failed oral antibiotics.

An infectious disease specialist evaluated him for a drug-resistant bacteria. The patient's original urine culture showed an extended-spectrum beta-lactamase, which meant that the usual antibiotics for a UTI would not have been effective. However, after reviewing the chart and prior cultures, I was not convinced that it was even causing an infection. Many previous urine cultures showed the same isolate, suggesting that it was colonizing the urinary tract . Colonization means that an organism resides on a tissue, such as the skin, urinary, and respiratory tracts, but does not cause an infection.

I contacted the care home and spoke with the nurse who knew him well. She informed me that he had increased confusion, and his urine was cloudier than usual and had an odor. Although a change in mental status can occur with infections, it happens periodically in someone with advanced dementia. Long-term catheters can harbor more resistant bacteria, which alone does not indicate an infection.

The nurse also mentioned that he had a few episodes of diarrhea the day of the transfer. After speaking with her, I reviewed the chart and examined the patient again. He had abdominal tenderness. The CT scan findings of nonspecific colonic wall thickening now made sense. I ordered a stool for *Clostridium difficile* PCR, which was positive and stopped the broad-spectrum antibiotic. He never did have a UTI. He began treatment for the *C. diff* and recovered promptly.

Collaboration in the Modern Medical Paradigm

In physician-to-physician collaboration, the openness of communication enriches patient care and improves physician job satisfaction. The case examples demonstrated how a breakdown could impact communication and quality of care. My decision to do more than was expected to the surgeon could be considered cavalier and disrespectful. The surgeon's avoidant response may have constituted unprofessionalism. Neither action was collaborative.

Collaboration has only become more challenging in the modern medical paradigm. Healthcare relies on increasing technology- and pharmaceutical-driven approaches. New therapies provide less invasive and more targeted options but complicate management. Consequently, to keep up with these advancements, patient care depends on the greater specialization of physicians.

Internal medicine is a specialty that has transformed over the years. There are now eleven recognized subspecialties, including pulmonary and critical care, endocrinology, infectious diseases, and rheumatology. Compounding this is a division in the continuity of care developed between inpatient stays and outpatient visits. In the nineties, the all-in-one provider went out of style and was no longer supportable. Time factors, pay schemes, increasingly complex patients, and the shift from private practice to hospital-based groups likely created a vacuum for a new job: full-time hospital doctor or hospitalist. Today, the paradigm of outpatient primary care doctors and hospitalists is the standard of care. In most studies, the quality of care is maintained or improved from the prior model (Goldman, 2003).

Technologies like electronic medical records have improved, allowing for greater ease of communication and collaboration, if not always in the most direct manner. Within hospital systems, interfaces exist for doctors to review a patient's records from the outpatient, inpatient, and outside hospitals. Improved smartphone storage and information transfer systems have given patients control of their medical information, a modern-day equivalent of a portable record booklet. Sometimes technology can help clarify the role of a practitioner and ease collaboration. However, a check-in phone call or visit may be required when findings are less clear.

Collaboration and communication retain their value in an increasingly fractured health care system. Although technology may enable information delivery and provide invaluable information, a solid doctor-patient relationship is the foundation of healthcare. Ultimately, the team must concentrate their efforts on fostering patient care. The next chapter will show how empathy and compassion are necessary ingredients for communication.

CHAPTER 9

Room for Empathy

Doctors are failing in matters of empathy and intuition, perhaps because of the present emphasis in diagnosis and therapy for 'evidence-based medicine,' based on measurable experience... Medicine in contemporary society may be failing because doctors do not listen to pleadings behind the spoken word.

-Philipp R, Philipp E, Thorne P.

Key Points

- Empathy, unlike sympathy, employs cognition and emotion. It provides a bridge that improves communication and better care and satisfaction between patients and physicians.

- Challenges to empathic listening include time constraints, compassion fatigue, and provider burnout.

- A physician applying interview techniques such as solicitation, framing, content reflection, and emotional calibration can maximize the doctor-patient interaction.

Case

Case 23: Empathy's Bridge

A physician might provide a patient with an effective service, but, at the same time, if the medical care lacks an empathic touch, something is not quite right. It is not "care" without human connection. A physician negotiates to stay on schedule or take the time to listen to patients and actively explore their emotions and concerns. Is there room for empathy in a busy practice? How does empathy enhance medical care? Will tomorrow's doctor be able to continue a practice rooted in compassion?

Empathy and initial patient visit

The initial clinic visit usually lasts from 40 to 60 minutes. This duration usually allows enough time to discuss a patient's health history. A physician can better understand the indications for each medication and have an opportunity to troubleshoot and discuss a patient's health goals. Occasionally, people will access the clinic for secondary gain. They may bring a list of their medications, some expired, hoping that a new doctor will prescribe them.

When meeting a new patient, it can sometimes be challenging to trust that they seek to improve their health. Some patients would instead take medications with side effects rather than face the discomfort of behavior change. However, sometimes even a glimmer of hope from an initial visit can start a chain reaction. It begins with an empathic connection.

Case 23: Empathy's Bridge

A 22-year-old woman came in seeking advice for her anxiety, which was at a point that it made it difficult for her to leave her house. After she discussed with me her feelings, I prompted her that I was going to ask about any significant childhood traumatic experiences. She mentioned that she witnessed parental abuse and had challenges coping with her parents' divorce.

She was running out of her medications and needed refills—another source of anxiety for her. She brought her boyfriend with her for moral support because it occasionally welled up during visits. The medicines included metformin and glyburide for her diabetes, lorazepam four times a day for anxiety disorder and post-traumatic stress disorder, hydrocodone for her neck pain, and inhalers for her asthma.

She provided me with information about her habits: she drank sugary drinks, alcohol, and smoked. When I asked her to estimate how much, she answered, "Twelve shots of whiskey daily." I asked her again, not comprehending the quantity, "Are you sure that is accurate?" She confirmed.

I asked whether she thought the alcohol could be triggering more anxiety. She was not aware of the effects of alcohol dependence. Her former provider told her to drink hard liquor instead of beer because it had fewer calories. Thus, she started medicating her anxiety with whiskey. I explained how alcohol could trigger anxiety after its effects wear off.

There were also severe risks with benzodiazepines and alcohol. I reviewed the medications and asked the patient to begin a course of medication reduction. I informed her to stop taking any of the "as-needed" meds. I agreed to work with her closely to assist her on a path to a healthy mind and body.

She returned for the next visit about a week later. I addressed the alcohol with her and asked her to consider a taper to avoid alcohol withdrawal from sudden cessation. I suggested she reduce her use by one shot of liquor every third day. In this circumstance, measuring it to be accurate was necessary. She brought in her calendar, showing me that she crossed off the completed days and wrote the number of shots. She proceeded along this path until she had stopped drinking her last nightly shot. She suffered a slight increase in anxiety, and she managed to create an outlet: walking in the park most days.

Once she stopped drinking alcohol and did not relapse for a few weeks, it was time to reduce the antianxiety medications. We talked about the risks of dose reduction. She took a relatively low dose of benzodiazepines but did it regularly—three to four tablets of 0.5mg lorazepam daily. Afterward, we began a slow taper off the lorazepam over the next several months.

With each reduction, she became successively more determined to quit. She realized that her mood swings were becoming less severe; she had fewer anxiety attacks. She thanked the clinic for the ease of contacting someone when she needed guidance and for the frequent visits. She was grateful for my support and clear instructions.

Empathy Defined

Empathy is a skill that combines cognition and emotion. It constructs a pathway to understanding another's feelings with a logical and emotional response. Unlike sympathy, where sentiments are shared, empathic clinicians share their *understanding* (Hojat, 2002). In the field of medicine, writers have described a "neutral empathy" or "detached concern" as if to de-emphasize the emotional aspect, which could affect objectivity (Blumgart, 1964). The term "clinical empathy" may resonate more than the seeming non sequitur "detached" or "neutral," again with the emphasis on understanding a patient's perspectives and reflecting on them (Hojat, 2002).

There is a different experience between knowing a patient's emotional state and acknowledging it to the patient. When physicians imagine themselves in "another's shoes" as they interact with a patient, a new realm of connection opens. This attunement allows the patient to feel comfortable, reduce stress, and reveal more to increase a physician's understanding (Halpern 2003).

In earlier chapters, I explained that words are translated in the brain both cognitively and emotionally. The brain interprets the words using their significance in prior experiences, applying various and unique meanings, both objective and subjective. For instance, the word "tumor" conveys tissue growth, benign or malignant. A patient might interpret this word as "cancer." Instead of asking a series of questions as a checklist or making statements, empathy opens the doorway into the patient's personal experience in processing the words. The physician may then take the critical step of checking back with the patient and offering clarification.

Awakening the "Heal" in Healthcare

When a patient enters the clinic, they seek to forge a relationship with a physician for the purpose of healing. Egnew described healing as "the personal experience of the transcendence of suffering" (Egnew, 2005). In practice, healing may have several meanings: discovering the source of the physical malady and providing a cure or an effective treatment if possible; reducing discomfort when cure is not possible; and empowering a person on their journey to health and positive change.

Although there is an inherent asymmetry in medical care, doctors can approach a patient with sensitivity and purpose for their benefit. Suppose the concerns, fears, and cues are neglected when a doctor addresses a patient's health issue. In that case, the physician compromises the quality of the dialogue and the fabric of the doctor-patient relationship.

Scott et al. developed the concept of a **Healing Relationship Model** between physician and patient, emphasizing the following elements: valuing relationships, appreciating power, and abiding. The model is nonjudgmental, fully immersed in the present moment, a practice of humility for the patient's benefit, and fosters a caring, developing relationship. The bridge of open dialogue allows the patient to receive optimal, tailored care. The physician garners information from a multifaceted perspective, not burdened by distrust or a hidden agenda. Both doctors and patients must explore these concerns; they become collaborators and partners at that moment. As a result, the members gain increasing trust, hope, and familiarity (Scott 2009).

Healing Relationship Model

- Valuing refers to listening and connecting without feeling that a patient is on an assembly line. It is not a quantity of time but a quality.

- Appreciating power occurs when a physician addresses that patient as a partner, inviting patients to consent, clarifying information, and making them aware of the options.

- Abiding relates to actions that a physician can take that show care and commitment to a patient.

Empathy and I-Thou

Is it acceptable for a physician to be a fine diagnostician but have a poor bedside manner? How about a doctor with an excellent bedside manner but limited clinical skills? Or for a surgeon to do excellent work but only focus on the surgical site and not reflect on the patient?

In his book *I and Thou*, the existentialist philosopher Martin Buber describes two potential relationship mindsets: *I -It* and *I-Thou*. The *I-Thou* interaction is a two-way exchange that exists without judgment or objectification, a meeting of subject-to-subject with a shared reality. An *I-it* encounter refers to how something is evaluated and deconstructed in a subject-to-object framework (Scott 2009). According to Buber, the *I-It* context, which in medicine includes scientific knowledge and procedures, provides value only as much as it occurs in the context of an *I-Thou* relationship, such as the doctor-patient relationship.

Medical care is replete with examples of *I-It* relationships. An ER physician reaches for a chart with a problem complaint of "drug overdose," and their colleague signs out to them about "the overdose in Room 11." A doctor orders a whole-body CT scan on a patient with a fever rather than clarifying the patient's history first. The patient's chart has several variables to check, including calculated kidney function, body mass index, and the parameters needed to enable higher coding. All of these do not function independently. They require the empathic connection of the *I-Thou*.

Approaching a person with an *I-It* relationship can lead to adverse outcomes. A doctor can treat a patient for shingles without factoring in their health history and give them three times the recommended dose of medication. A radiologist may only clue in on the worst-case scenarios of a CT scan ordered for "chest pain," such as an aneurysm or pneumothorax, yet miss the air under the diaphragm. A nurse may deliver a lethal dose of insulin because she followed the order without checking back with the physician. In each of these errors, the objective findings were not enough when devoid of context. The person for whom these studies and treatments are prescribed gives it a context.

Barriers to Empathy

Compassion fatigue, or empathy fatigue, results from a flood of clinical demands that require attention and empathic listening. A consequence of fatigue is increased stress, sometimes to the point of traumatizing the professional (Figley, 1995). Exhaustion may develop when compassion channels sympathy, "feeling with" rather than empathy, "feeling into." Stepping out to gain perspective, a person who empathizes still does not lose themselves in the process.

On the other hand, sympathy is a place of sharing pain rather than acknowledging it. A person mentalizes the patient's experience of pain and suffering and attempts to understand it by imagining that they had it (Thirioux, 2016). Conceivably, sympathy could hinder one from viewing the turmoil objectively and free of bias. As we will see in the next chapter, the antidote for empathy fatigue is self-compassion, self-care, and mindfulness.

Physician burnout, or professional exhaustion, results from an imbalance of demand and achievement and exerts pressure on a physician, leading to ongoing stress and demoralization. Burnout manifests as **depersonalization**, not considering humanity in other people, and **withdrawal**. As the degree of burnout worsens, empathic connections become hindered. Interestingly, physicians and other healthcare workers with higher empathy levels have greater satisfaction and less burnout (Sturzu, 2019; Taleghani, 2017). Does empathy positively affect both physicians and patients to explain this? Does the physician gain job satisfaction by reducing a patient's anxiety and improving clinical outcomes?

Time factors are a frequent concern and a barrier to empathic listening. Physicians sometimes leverage time for empathy during a visit. They must let go of the prior visit and other distractors at the door and enter the room to be receptive to another person. Expressing empathy does not require much time. When physicians try to keep a fast pace or fall behind schedule, the priority of time overtakes that of listening. The physician finds themselves making quick judgments and assumptions; neither of these is always accurate.

Think of what happens when the lead guitar is out of tune with the rest of the instruments. The whole song suffers no matter how nice the drums, the bass, and the singer's voice sound. Likewise, physician burnout hinders empathic attunement and detrimentally affects both patient and provider. Making room for empathy boosts the quality of patient care, and physicians also benefit from the exchange.

I once saw an established patient who came in late for his yearly check-up, and seeing him meant that I would have to skip my lunch. He had a history of a heart attack in his mid-forties (ten years before) and periodically saw his cardiologist. He would bring his labs and cardiologist's notes for each visit, speak a few stilted words, and leave as if checking off an assignment. When I saw him, I decided to press him further, asking him whether he was trying to improve his health or just do the bare minimum. When I persisted, he showed discomfort and declared, "I don't think I want you as my doctor anymore." I apologized for the way I asked him, not intending to make it an interrogation of his intentions. Although I attempted to motivate him, it only came off as shaming because I did not approach him with empathy and active listening skills. I was not in tune with him, and it alienated him. The interaction left an indelible impression on me about the importance of compassionate listening and a patient-centered approach.

Empathy in a Busy Practice

Empathic connection is not only beneficial but necessary. Both the patient and physician ensure that they listen with inclusion and partnership. Quality of care, patient satisfaction, and patient understanding flow from the perspectives that this partnership allows. A patient may signal a "call" to connect with a statement or question. These often come as short invitations for a physician to recognize and respond in as little as one sentence or even a few words. One study, which analyzed patient visits for empathic opportunities, determined that physicians only responded to about 10 percent of empathic opportunities and, if so, in the final third of the visit (Morse 2008). Moreover, this study was about patient visits for lung cancer—a particularly sensitive theme.

How can a doctor participate in an empathic connection in a fifteen-minute visit? An awareness that words often emanate from emotional pathways is a good start. Remember that empathy is a skill that acknowledges a patient's emotions and meets them at that place, even if briefly. A physician can observe the words and the signals that accompany them: the specific choice of words or phrases, word repetition or stuttering, and nonverbal cues such as sighs, facial movements, or body posturing. Questions from the patient are often initial cues.

A physician can respond as an active listener to questions and statements with a simple recognition of the patient's possible state of mind. The language must be expressed clearly and with a tone of reflection. A brief response with just a few words or statements can often affirm that a physician understands and is present with the patient's emotional experience.

A provider can employ the following tools (Coulehan 2001):

- **Active Listening** includes verbal and nonverbal cues to listening, as discussed in Chapter 7. It requires that a physician focuses on the patient's narrative while providing them with an open platform to communicate.

• **Framing** is a way to clarify understanding, as physicians ensure their words capture the patient's narrative. Before framing the patient's words, the physician may say, "I am going to make sure that I have this right…."

• **Content reflection** merges the patient's statement with the patient's feelings and concerns. An example of a thought might be, "Sounds like you are concerned that your dizziness may represent a more serious problem."

• **Emotional calibration** allows a physician to understand the gravity of a patient's situation or concerns with their emotional response to it. They may feel fearful, angry, or sad. Identifying the emotion can improve trust in the exchange. "Tell me how this makes you feel."

• **Soliciting**. Sometimes, the information is not complete. Physicians can ask for clarification and correction to understand the patient's story clearly. "Is there anything I missed?"

How a physician addresses a patient is crucial. It can ebb and flow from one encounter to another because of workflow, life stressors, and a physician's unmet self-care needs. A patient may be viewed as a total being or just a "problem list." Most people would not see the latter as empathic. It does not take extra time to exercise empathy. A physician with these skills opens the gates to improved patient care and career satisfaction.

The greatest mistake in the treatment of diseases is that there are physicians for the body and physicians for the soul, although the two cannot be separated.

—Plato

CHAPTER 10

On Burnout and Creating Resilience

Key Points

• The ingredients of burnout include depersonalization, lack of efficacy, and exhaustion.

• Consequences of burnout include increased provider turnover, risk of medical errors, decreased patient support, and job dissatisfaction.

• Physicians and other providers can approach burnout by engendering open discussion and a group support culture. Large healthcare corporations can actively support their employees by creating workshops, questionnaires, and a culture that upholds quality patient care and physician support rather than bottom-line finances.

• Providers can develop resilience and protection against burnout through self-compassion and self-care practices, workload reduction, volunteering, mindfulness meditation, hobby development, and non-clinical practices.

Being a physician can tax health, relationships, and free time. I remember how much weight I gained through residency. There were too many weddings I could not go to because of my work schedule. I cannot relive all the smiles and giggles I missed on the faces of my young children because of staying late at work. As I write this book, I wonder if setting a better work-life balance as a priority would have protected my marriage from the strain it went through because of the work demands.

The truth is that burnout results from placing duties, expectations, and workplace stressors over a physician's personal needs. Although the cause of this may not be directly within a physician's control, the responsibility to address burnout lies in a concerted effort of health organizations, physician groups, and the culture of medicine. Fortunately, there are some things that every student, resident, and physician can do to protect from burnout and rekindle the creative flow that all of us would benefit from having. Starting in medical school, students can equip themselves with support systems, healthy practices, and other skills that build resilience.

Clinical medicine is a service-oriented field. A physician may begin with an unfettered altruistic spirit. Over time, these ideals can gradually erode with real-life experiences, greater responsibility, and longer hours. Each day, a physician engages with a flood of patient concerns, conditions, requests, and challenges. Managing authorities evaluate a practice by its ability to meet cold parameters such as waiting time, patients seen, income generated, and other metrics and not as often on the collaborative skill, passion for the field, love of teaching, or clinical prowess. A physician may become tainted with skepticism and worn by the many years of long shifts, a web of increased responsibilities (work creep), and limited autonomy. Sometimes it is enough to cause a physician to face work hardships or even leave the practice.

Physician burnout refers to a long-term stress response characterized by emotional fatigue and a negative attitude. It is prevalent in medical practice. In a survey conducted by Medscape, as many as 46 percent of physicians reported burnout, almost one in two physicians. Burnout reduces morale, increases the risk for errors, and leads to depersonalization, relationship strain, and even drug abuse and suicide.

Although I did not think it was at the time, the increasing workload instigated burnout in me. After experiencing work demoralization in my life, I have become more aware of ways to prevent it and stay resilient. I have also become more proactive in discussing work-life balance and witnessing burnout risk factors in my colleagues.

My Journey to Understanding Burnout

I rotated in the intensive care unit (ICU) twice annually during my residency. The physician coverage consisted of three teams, alternating calls every third night.[61] In the ICU, the workload was just as intensive. We often faced sleep deprivation and endless nights. The fatigue dragged into the next day. We frequently worked well into the post-call days to complete all our duties before leaving home somewhat in a daze. Although this was quite a strain, it was encapsulated in one month. In residency, we constantly reminded each other that even the worst night of call would end, and so too, the most brutal rotation months.

Physician burnout does not just end after taking a vacation or when the workload decreases. My experience with burnout gradually developed over the years as an attending. I saw a large panel of patients with multiple chronic conditions in an outpatient setting. Initially, I could not find a full-time infectious disease position moving out west, so I agreed to work on a hybrid inpatient infectious disease with outpatient primary care. I welcomed the change. The first eight months were a honeymoon period, with enough gaps in the schedule to keep it running smoothly. In time, my patient panel grew. Through the following year, the daily schedule became more frequently full. Patients called to be seen sooner, and multiple faxes and orders showed up on my desk to sign. At first, this was manageable. And, for my fatigue, a strategically placed vacation went a long way to replenish my energy.

Enter the electronic health records (EHR) system. Perfunctory tasks previously delegated to medical assistants fell into my bucket to complete, along with seeing patients and updating their records. Providers received no additional time to complete the chart tasks. The daily schedule and visit times remained twenty minutes for follow-ups and forty minutes for new patients. A physician requires extra time for each visit to complete the Electronic Health Record. Charting extended shorter visits by ten minutes and comprehensive visits by twenty minutes.

The workload led to a snowball effect on my schedule, which ate into my lunch hour, often not permitting me to take time for myself. In the second half of the day, the time I needed to complete records caused me to stay past clinic hours, racing to get things done and get home on time for dinner. After putting the kids to bed in the evening, I went through the numerous remaining lab results, patient messages, and requests from care homes, sometimes the same material included in duplicates or triplicates.

Work piled up, often requiring an extra two to three hours a night. EHRs show a list of tasks to complete, including calls from care facilities, patient calls, lab results, and medication renewals. I seldom got the list below one hundred tasks. To make matters worse, even after working several hours a night, the number would shoot up by sixty new requests daily. I struggled with working a few hours every evening or taking a night off, only to face a heavier load the next day. The exhaustion built up. I grew a deeper understanding of how it felt to be Sisyphus[62].

I frequently faced the decision to either get a good sleep or do more charting, often choosing the latter. My body signaled that it was being challenged with physical conditions, including nerve pain issues from chronic upper back and neck strain, bulging cervical discs, and carpal tunnel syndrome.

My story was not unlike other doctors in the clinic. One of our new physicians had even more leftover tasks each day. She was an excellent physician with outstanding interpersonal communication skills and a solid knowledge base. I often commiserated with her on the futility of having no tasks in the buckets while secretly feeling relieved that my situation was not as dire as hers.

We were among the many physicians who grappled with the new role of "perfunctory technician." No one could imagine that, after medical training, a doctor would need more time to complete computer tasks than provide patient care. One study found that *the average physician spends about two hours on the EHR for every one hour of direct patient care!* For each patient, the time it takes for documentation extends an office visit by 6.3%, but it decreases the patient time by 8.5% (Jourkes, 2018). Additionally, doctors may spend one to two hours of personal time working into the night (Sinsky, 2016).

The administration met with us and advised us to code higher (up-code)[63] and see more patients. We could even get a bonus if we met Relative Value Unit (RVU) benchmarks. What was not discussed was that up-coding would require more chart documentation, and seeing more patients meant more results, calls, and interfacing with the EHR. It became a choice between quality of life or "golden handcuffs."

In my case, the business end was not sensitive to the general quality of life over financial incentives; they flexed the ability to hire another "body" if we were dissatisfied with these options. It became apparent that our interests were secondary to how we could profit the company or, at the very least, reduce the revenue hemorrhage prevalent in primary care. Physicians started to leave the practice.

What are RVUs?

The magic numbers, that medical administration too often focus on, are the number of patients seen and procedures. They calculate productivity indices, such as Relative Value Units (RVU) to compare physician output. The RVU is a composite number which factors in patient work, practice expenses, and professional liability insurance costs (Katz, 2016). Physicians who see patients in the outpatient setting require longer visits, and, consequently, have lower RVUs than those that perform procedures like surgery or endoscopy.

Consequently, to meet RVU incentives, outpatient physicians may see more patients. Challenges include reductions in Medicare compensation, increased patient complexity, and lack of procedural or other office services. Administrations may incentivize physicians to increase their work-related RVUs by seeing more patients. They may not recognize that the increase in workload can further strain physicians and compromise quality of care.

As I continued working in that setting, I often reflected on my initial decision to become a doctor. I imagined a young physician with ideals and a thirst for knowledge discovering the reality that medicine can become: a respected, service-oriented vocation transforming into a lackluster, unfulfilling job. I aspired to be a skilled servant to my patients, but the work shifted to a stale job devoid of creative freedom. This experience was a feeling of something missing, a lack of efficacy.

After spending hours each day completing tasks, the patients themselves can even become tasks. This is what is meant by the term depersonalization. Both patients and doctors suffer because of it. Compounded by this work strain was the fear of missing something lost in the minutia of tasks, something for which I would be held responsible.

Ingredients of physician burnout include **depersonalization**, **lack of efficacy**, and **exhaustion**— I had all three of them. After six years of working in the same clinic, I decided it was time for me to either quit medicine or drastically change my practice setting. I resigned. Initially, I was ambivalent because I treasured the relationships with my established patients. My departure would mean that they would have to find a new physician. I realized that I had to prioritize my needs to be an effective doctor to any patient.

The three-month notice was not soon enough after all the years of chart work. Was I burned out or just ready to move on? Probably both. My colleague took a quick exit after working at the clinic for less than a year. I know, like me, she missed her patients greatly, but that was not as crucial as unmet personal needs. If physicians compromise self-care, how can they be compassionate to others? I factored this into the plans that I would make for my next career move. I would happily accept less pay for greater autonomy and another chance to care for patients.

Would doctors pick better pay or an improved quality of life?

Quality of life won over pay. More than half of the fifteen thousand doctors surveyed voted for a $20,000 salary reduction to reduce work hours (Medscape, 2020). For most physicians, work-life balance ranks on top, while compensation places a distant second (48% vs. 23% in men, 42% vs. 16% in women) (Medscape, 2021).

The Root Cause of Physician Burnout

One way of looking at burnout is that it signifies a *stressed system.* The term *burnout syndrome* may be more apt because it describes a condition that results from chronic stress from a mismatch between a physician and the work environment (Montero-Marin, 2009). Burnout comprises three dimensions: exhaustion, depersonalization or cynicism, and loss of professional efficacy (Maslach, 1996). Burnout occurs in any occupation. Although there may be an overlap between burnout and depression or anxiety, these conditions are separate entities (Koutsimani, 2019).

The 3 Elements of Burnout

- Depersonalization
- Lack of Efficacy
- Exhaustion

Farber proposed additional specifiers to further characterize burnout and allude to more targeted approaches: **frenetic** (increased workload), **under-challenged** (monotony from an insufficient workload), and **worn out** (stress-load and decreased gratification) (Farber, 1990). In retrospect, the increased workload and type of work challenged me as I strained to maintain quality while completing tasks in a system that provided no relief.

Healthcare quality has become compromised in the era of electronic medical records, decreased compensation, and increased medical complexity. At one time, physicians had more autonomy when private practice was the usual model. As care became more specialized and intensive, smaller hospitals could not stay afloat without financial collaboration from large health systems. These systems acquired many private practices, as there were increasingly greater overhead costs.

Large companies commonly run medical care all too often with financial bottom lines. Revenue generation competes with the provision of quality healthcare. Physicians become cogwheels instead of collaborators, which devalues both patients and physicians. Apathy and decreased morale follow. Fortunately, there is a silver lining with new models factoring in quality metrics, emphasizing value over volume. Value-based care may temper production-centered compensation models and support primary care physicians. (Keegan, 2013). Focusing on physician well-being and de-emphasizing productivity benefits physicians and organizations. Losing a physician could result in high costs of lost revenue, recruitment, training, and practice-building (Shanafelt, 2017).

Dike Drummond, an expert on burnout and physician himself, likens it to negative balances on physical, emotional, and spiritual energy accounts. Although physicians can still function in a depleted state, the work ripples into personal life, influencing relationships, efficacy, and larger questions on life's purpose. Drummond asks physicians to protect their energy accounts "you can't give (as a provider) what you don't have." A physician may consider several options: from least risky to most, to fit in the constructs of the current system; to take a measured risk and try another location; to reinvent their career; and to get out of medicine (Drummond, 2015).

Surveys consistently show that about 1 in 2 physicians have signs of burnout. Physicians in the fields of critical care (51%), rheumatology (50%), and infectious diseases (49%) reported the highest rates (Medscape, 2021.) Although burnout rates were high during the COVID-19, many physicians, nurses, and other healthcare workers reported experiencing burnout before the pandemic began (Sullivan, 2022).

What causes burnout, and why is it particularly prevalent in physicians and other caregivers? One reason for burnout is that it is intrinsic to being a caregiver, seeing patients who have fears, worries, and suffering, along with diagnostic and care challenges. *Interestingly, doctors, nurses, social workers, and teachers all have high rates of burnout. They all provide service to others.*

The Consequences of Physician Burnout

Aside from the turmoil burnout can place on an individual physician's life, such as the need to find a new job, concerns about efficacy, spiraling out of control with substance use, and increased suicidal ideation, burnout can affect the very system that provoked it. One symptom of physician burnout is **turnover**. As I discovered personally, starting in a new practice after leaving an old one comes with a honeymoon period. It begins, almost uncomfortably, with many open slots in the schedule and evolves over the next several months to become saturated with appointments.

After about a year, as the panel grows, visits are scheduled and filled out for several weeks, increasing the demand for a patient to be double-booked to be seen sooner. Compounding this is that a busier schedule increases workload as more patients get bloodwork, study results, and request calls. One day the physician may discover that they are in the same place in the new setting as in the old, with the same ingredients for burnout: expectations, demand, and work creep.

On the other side of turnover are the loss of physician personnel and the severing of doctor patient relationships. I was in a small group practice in a rural area that lost one or two doctors every year. Physicians did not readily fill these absent positions. Consequently, this meant that the remaining doctors would assume the patient panel of the departed doctor. Physician turnover increased work on those who remained, further straining the system.

Meanwhile, patients must decide whether they want to stay in the same clinic and face starting a new physician relationship. The visits come at the cost of compromising the stream of open patient communication as they adjust to the new provider's practice style and wonder if they could leave too. Physician turnover was associated with measurable decreases in **patient satisfaction** ratings and the likelihood of getting care quickly (Reddy, 2015).

COVID-19 and Burnout

The COVID-19 pandemic has been a catalyst for change in many people. Health guidelines prioritized public safety over other practices, including clinic visits, social activities, worship, and school. The world waited for COVID-19 to pass, a shared experience in time but not in space, as countries and regions were affected differently. It became apparent that it was not just going to disappear suddenly.

The pandemic put burnout and work fatigue at the forefront. In a survey conducted in February 2021, more than half of respondents felt burned out, and two-thirds believed burnout had worsened during the pandemic. Another study of 18,935 nurses during the COVID-19 pandemic showed that 34% felt emotionally exhausted, 12.6% had depersonalization, and 15% felt a lack of accomplishment—all elements of burnout (Galanis, 2021).

The experience of burnout does not occur from a lack of mental strength, and it does not melt away by taking a vacation. Organizations are often ill-equipped to address these challenges or provide additional support to their workforces. Although we are just beginning to realize the mass exodus of nurses from traditionally paid hospital positions, the lack of staffing has had severe ramifications for patient care. Consider New York City, a city with high rates of COVID cases; there was a 400% increase in nurses looking for new jobs in 2020.

The situation was so dire that the US Bureau of Labor Statistics reported that the inpatient healthcare workforce was down 524,000 jobs since February 2020, the brunt of lost work in nursing and residential care facilities. The pandemic has exposed long-standing workforce shortages in nursing, which were already short-staffed before COVID.

Addressing Burnout and Resilience

Physician employment is the raison d'être for health organizations, in which physicians generate income from patient visits, referrals for diagnostic studies, and procedures. Like in any work environment, when a job is not conducive to change, the physician may *exit* (leaving the job or the profession) or *give voice* (negotiate, protest, complain) (Kravitz, 2012). If a physician is discontent and leaves a job, they may have made an individual correction, but the disagreeable work environment continues for those who remain. Nevertheless, resigning may not always be necessary. Physicians have considerable leverage in negotiating and bargaining their work arrangements, salaries, and expectations. They may identify factors causing stagnation or instigating physician demoralization and offer creative approaches for the administration.

The Shift in Reimbursement Models: Value-based health care

The health system is fractured. Most spending (90%) goes to medical care, while preventive efforts go largely unaddressed. Currently, 60 percent of the US population has one or more chronic conditions, including obesity, high blood pressure, and diabetes (Rand, 2017.)

Sometimes not of their own volition, doctors prioritize damage control over partnering with patients to address behavior and restore health. Health administrators' pressures to meet quotas, patient satisfaction scores, electronic health records, and computerized order entry exacerbate physician burnout. Physicians who genuinely treasure doctor-patient relationships and compassionate practices are left astray by these demands.

In the era of multiple stakeholders in healthcare, both physicians and patients suffer from unmet expectations. **Value-based health care** is an attempt to improve a patient's experience, address a population's health needs, and reduce health care costs (Teisbert, 2019.) The framework factors patient outcomes with expenses, or "the best bang for the health care buck" (Tsevat, 2018).

Value-based care focuses on the three "c's" of patient aims: *capability*, *comfort*, and *calm*. Care should prioritize value while restoring a patient's health (capability and comfort) and allow them to continue to live their usual way as they receive care (calm) (Wallace, 2016). This approach may restore the physician's role as a healer by emphasizing value over other productivity models. Proponents cite that these measures also encourage empathy and reduce provider burnout (Teisbert, 2019.)

Taking Back the Power

Burnout rates in medicine are high, supporting that all students and physicians should consider the factors that increase their risk of burnout. Knowledge is power, and the Maslach Burnout Inventory (MBI) can identify if you may already be developing burnout[64]. With proper attention, a provider may be able to protect themselves from more significant ramifications of burnout, including medical errors, job loss, and depression.

Ultimately, physicians are more than a company's job statement. One helpful exercise is to reverse the concept of a job description.

Instead of looking at job opportunities and their characteristics and reviewing the numbers, what if you could construct your job? What kind of practice would you build if you had complete autonomy and no financial strain? Now write out your job description. For tomorrow's doctors, it is a reminder that we can set the pace and schedule in our careers after training.

Here is a similar question for the general audience: how would you use the time in your life if you followed your calling? The answer is unique for each person and affected by timing and circumstances. It could be a hybrid of various responsibilities for physicians, each balancing out the other. It may be a job that stimulates interest, provides service to others, and is collegial. It would be work that someone is excited to wake up and get started. For me, it incorporates my interests and writing goals, a chance to instruct students and residents, travel for speaking and conference activities, and sufficient time for each patient visit to allow for a robust physician-patient relationship and a thorough evaluation. Although these questions are commonly considered in a physician desiring to downshift before retirement, they should be the standard review for a physician at any stage in their career.

The seeds of burnout may begin early in a physician's career, as they become indoctrinated in medicine's work ethic and culture. As many as 50 percent of medical students and residents have already reported feeling burnout during their training (Dyrbye, 2014.) Lacking in the culture of medicine is an open dialogue of issues that fuel burnout within the physician community.

The field of medicine espouses self-sacrifice, compassion, and altruism, all of which are honorable traits. However, much too often, physicians-in-training are inculcated with perfectionism, prioritizing work, minimal self-care, and keeping stress inside instead of the messages of humility, professionalism, and self-compassion (Shanafelt, 2019). Without a framework, the individual physicians often must cope and make survival changes to protect themselves from burnout, sometimes with the not-so-healthy "work hard, play hard mentality ."

On July first of each year, a medical student transitions abruptly into an intern. This day marks the beginning of rigorous residency training, often filled with long hours and many patients. A typical day combines the didactic hours of the morning report, noon conference, and the usual duties of patient care and team rounds. The end of the day comes when the intern completes their patient care, notes, and orders—sometimes after an evening of call. As an intern, this could mean an extended post-call day since sleep deprivation slows down work efficiency the next day. I recall how I would uncontrollably nap in between writing the patient notes and orders post-call. I feared making a mistake in the hospital or getting into a car accident by falling asleep at the wheel after hospital duties.

On Culture Change in Medicine: Out with the old and in with the new?

In 2003, residency programs issued changes on trainee work shifts for improved wellbeing, quality of care, and patient safety. These efforts were promulgated by the American College of Graduate Medical Education (ACGME) and called for caps on work weeks (80 hours) and consecutive hours worked (16 hours for interns and 24 hours for residents).

The precedent to residency work hour restrictions was New York state, which enacted Rule 405.4 in July 1989. The law resulted from a civil suit regarding possible negligent care of Libby Zion brought against New York Hospital by Libby's parents. Although the cause of Libby's death was not directly related to her care[65], the case led to the formation of statewide restrictions on residency programs. A group of academic physicians referred to as the Bell Commission made recommendations that appear in the 405.4 rule: these include an 80-hour workweek cap, no more than 24 consecutive hours of work, and on-call and post-call policies to manage the workloads (Kramer, 2010).

A common criticism at the time, especially with older attendings, was the idea of "when I was a resident…" as they described longer days and more night calls. These physicians raised concerns that fewer hours could mean more learning gaps and less endurance. These complaints overlooked the cost of medical errors, demoralization, and the harm of sleep deprivation. Neuroscience findings support getting sufficient sleep to allow the brain time to consolidate new information and retain what was learned (Diakelmann, 2010).

A transformative shift in the culture of medicine brings with it the positive ideals of the profession while emphasizing collaborative efforts of communication and physician support. Edgar Schein refers to the changes as "managed evolution," or fine-tuning of the culture, adopting new beliefs while discarding others (Schein, 2010). Patient care benefits too when physicians address their needs in a supportive culture.

Physicians can also drive the cultural shift in decisions regarding their professional goals. Many may assume that the current model of care works well enough. Others might be concerned about burning bridges in changing out a typical physician job for something less predictable. Furthermore, medical schools have not taught resilience lessons until recently. These skills can also be learned through residency and attending physician training programs.

Work-life Balance and Developing Resilience

Why work toward an ideal work-life balance? I asked myself that question. My answer was to start from a blank slate and work several jobs. I found infectious diseases jobs where I could work three days a week; I added a public health consultant job weekly; this meant I had about a day and a half for writing and education time. Once I removed the burden of clerical tasks, I could reframe each day as an opportunity to provide support to patients and physicians rather than a job that pays the bills. I also found time to write, start a health information blog, and publish books. I have never looked back.

Resilience relates to growth and adaptation, even in the setting of adversity or dilemma. Physicians who wield resilience buffer themselves from burnout triggers in medical practice. The rigors of medical training equip the physician with a degree of fortitude. However, physician resilience programs provide an opportunity to expand skills that reduce burn-out risk. The best programs involve the health care institutions in which physicians are employed rather than solely physician-driven programs (Epstein, 2013).

Counter to the enculturation and adaptation that stokes burnout, physicians can learn resilience skills and play an instrumental role in directing their future practice. The goal of resilience training is to allow time for self-reflection and self-care and to develop skills for managing work-related stress (Cordova et al., 2020). These programs consist of small-group instruction and shared experience. In a randomized clinical trial, these programs effectively decreased the rates of depersonalization (15.5 percent less vs. 0.8 percent control), emotional exhaustion, and overall burnout. They were sustainable 12 months after the study (West, 2020).

Alternative approaches could include career-long exposures, beginning in medical school, and selecting topics based on the career stage of the physician. One example of a physician resilience program is a year-long, voluntary course on mindfulness practices, narrative medicine, and stress management training. Shorter interventions, like one-day workshops or online training modules, are unlikely to be as impactful as longer-term approaches (Cordova, 2020).

Another essential factor for physician well-being is a positive work environment. The practice of medicine has become an increasingly insular experience, with more work required for electronic medical records. Although multiple physicians may be in one practice, their busy schedules can sometimes conflict with developing an environment of collegiality and community. Physicians in the same practice may benefit from blocking time to meet regularly as a community to voice concerns and offer support. Workplace settings could also consider implementing methods to reduce inefficient practices, ensure appropriate staffing, and survey physicians for potential challenges before they intensify.

Self-Awareness and Self-Care

Growth and resilience relate to **Chapters 2** and **3** on behavior and bias. In the setting of work stresses, physicians may choose to address the situation in front of them and sideline self-care. An over-extended physician may ignore the early signs of burnout. **Self-awareness** of one's responses to stress through mindfulness approaches, such as meditation and skills training, can equip physicians with greater sensitivity to direct their future practice. **Self-care** support is also paramount, such as exercise, meditation, relaxation techniques, proper sleep, and minimizing distractions (e.g., smartphone time).

What originates as a physician grappling with workplace challenges, increasing patient demands, and the ever-present EHR task extends to adverse patient outcomes, poor workplace morale, and physician attrition. Imagine applying the life lesson taught in an airplane, "put on your mask before assisting someone else," but only the plane has a faulty overhead mask compartment. In a malignant workplace environment, self-care efforts can be equally challenging, even for those well-prepared.

Physicians must communicate their needs, calibrate clinical responsibilities with personal ones, set limits, and prioritize self-care. However, with such a high prevalence of burnout, or workplace demoralization, in medical practice, we are reminded that it is a product of a system that too commonly emphasizes what a physician can produce rather than the quality they provide to it (Gabel, 2013). Physician morale is nurtured in the context of a proactive health system that bolsters its providers, creates a fertile environment for the community, and encourages collaborative and creative problem-solving.

Burnout-Proof Interventions for Physicians to Become Resilient and Inspired

Sometimes a person must endure a challenge to learn to protect themselves from it in the future. We are talking about knowledge gained through personal experience. I want to provide an opportunity for *fortuitous learning*, or knowledge gained through someone else's experience, so that physicians may benefit no matter where they are in their career. There is no silver bullet that targets the nascent development of burnout. What is certain is that if a physician is developing burnout, it will not go away on its own without an action plan.

Several strategies may be helpful to protect medical students, residents, or physicians from burnout or mitigate the challenges to those who have thought about leaving the profession. These include time factors, such as time management skills and workload reduction, taking time to volunteer locally or internationally, changing to a non-clinical career in medicine, or developing other hobbies or a "side gig."

1. Time Factors: Time Management and Workload Reduction

The way we spend time in the day dramatically impacts our well-being. In a recent survey, the two critical contributors to burnout were "too many bureaucratic tasks" and "spending too many hours at work" (Peckman, 2017). If burnout occurs from the excessive demands of a busy clinic or hospital job, what would happen if physicians reduced their workload? A study found a correlation between burnout and increased workload; autonomy predicted a lower likelihood (Shirom, 2009). For some individuals experiencing burnout, no abbreviated schedule would address what they are going through. Also, a reduced plan may not seem immediately attainable for others because of their current job arrangement. After all, a high workload is typical among physicians. In a Medscape survey, 28% of physicians reduced work hours to address burnout (Medscape, 2021).

2. Mindfulness Practices

Your Health Forum strongly supports mindfulness meditation (MM) and other relaxation practices. They can help reduce burnout in medical staff too. An analysis of sixteen papers on MM and its use on nursing students suggested a positive impact, including stress, anxiety, depression, and burnout (van der Riet, 2018). Aside from traditional mindfulness practices, proper sleep, regular exercise, and daily downtime and stress management techniques contribute to greater resilience to depression, anxiety, and burnout.

Interestingly, mindfulness meditation increases gray matter in the frontal cortex and other areas of the brain that correlate with learning, cognition, memory, and empathy. Importantly, these changes can occur over a brief period . Another way to look at it is that resilience develops through learning and promotes structural brain changes.

3. Shared Dialogue and Social Support

The stigma attached to burnout often allows nascent issues to grow until they become too large to go unnoticed. Yet many hospital administrators are ill-equipped to manage burnout proactively, frequently finding themselves in high turnover situations when these issues go unaddressed. Mindful communication through shared dialogue can help address both ingredients of burnout: mismatched expectations and unspoken concerns.

Communication and social support address suppressed emotions and allow healing and problem-solving to replace the isolation that comes with burnout. One beneficial program with a hospital system I worked for was a Commensality group that met monthly over dinner, funded by the hospital system. A Commensality group[66] is an evidence-based model to improve cohesiveness and collegiality among doctors in a practice setting. The meetings consist of 6-8 physicians and are held once monthly over coffee or dinner for a minimum of 6 months. In my group, we talked about work-life issues and burnout prevention strategies, as we listened to and supported one another.

Medical practices that hold workshops for their staff can improve well-being and protect against burnout. A study of seventy physicians in NY showed that training programs, amounting to an all-day session and ten monthly 2.5-hour sessions, impacted job satisfaction and buffered physicians from demoralization. There was also a benefit in empathy, something that often suffers in the setting of physician burnout (Krasner, 2009).

4. Volunteerism and International Humanitarian Work

While volunteer and missionary burnout does occur, sometimes changing their work scenery can benefit someone experiencing these challenges. It can help physicians rediscover the joy of providing care and create a new narrative as they return to their work setting. There may be less emphasis on medical charting, the number of patients seen, and time spent with each patient— elements that exacerbate burnout. Whether a physician volunteers in a developing country or a local free clinic, they realize the rewards of working in a community that requires and appreciates assistance.

When I applied to medical school, I felt a calling to volunteer in developing countries. It was strong enough to investigate taking a gap year and delaying the start. I decided to incorporate international training and volunteerism starting in medical school. The first experience was a five-week trip to Kenya organized by a fellow student from a village near Lake Victoria. The stark contrast in Kenya's culture and life experience versus the comforts that I took for granted in the United States left an impression on me.

Something as simple as turning on the faucet to fill a glass with potable water may take more than a half hour's hike in rural Kenya and other parts of the world. The WHO and UNICEF estimate that more than a quarter of the global population does not have access to clean water and must fetch water elsewhere (WHO & UNICEF, 2017). The implications on health and sanitation, work productivity, education, and leisure time, particularly for the women and girls usually tasked with this job, are enormous (UNICEF, 2016). Within developing countries, diarrhea from drinking contaminated water remains a leading cause of death[67] in children under five worldwide (UNICEF, 2021).

International humanitarian work early in training can put things into context. It enhanced my confidence in the history and physical examination components and reinforced my commitment to quality and empathic care. I have enjoyed taking time away from home throughout my career to volunteer in countries such as Haiti, Guatemala, and Lesotho. A short trip out of one's comfort zone can increase fulfillment and bolster adaptability, people skills, and resilience — all valuable skills to prevent burnout (Kolkin, 2018).

5. Mentorship

Medical training takes the form of an apprenticeship, where experienced physician mentors teach mentees, ideally in an individualized and supportive fashion. Even the title "Doctor" comes from the Latin *docēre*, meaning "to teach." My mentors were instrumental to my training, serving as educators and role models. As trainees transition from students to doctors, they too can actively participate in mentoring those earlier in their training (Platz, 2013).

For medical students, an effective mentoring program improves personal accomplishment, one of the contributors to burnout when lacking (Jordan, 2019). In a peer nursing mentorship study, where fourth-year students mentored first-years, internal locus of control (LOC) was higher after participation (Demir, 2014). Locus of control relates to an individual's perspective of a stressor and their ability to address it. Someone with an external LOC believes that circumstances are not changeable; someone with an internal LOC takes greater responsibility for managing a stressor and effective coping.

I spent my career in various capacities as a mentor for medical students. Each year, I accepted third- and fourth-year medical students for rotations with me in infectious diseases or primary care. Although the time spent teaching makes the day a little longer, it is stimulating to interact with students and a terrific way to "pay it forward" and train future doctors. I recently ran into a student who rotated with me years ago and now practices family medicine. I was delighted to learn that she still reflects on the time she trained with me. A commitment to mentorship can create a sense of efficacy and restore job satisfaction.

6. Non-clinical Practice

Medical school and residency training provide highly sought-after perspectives for non-clinical positions. These jobs include working as a consultant, educator, and supervisor, including writing and editing. It might just be what the doctor ordered (ha!). In a survey of ninety-five nonclinical faculty who answered the Abbreviated Maslach Burnout Inventory, only 1% of respondents reported high burnout, and 35% percent said a medium amount (Ofei-Dodoo, 2018). These rates of burnout are much lower than clinical providers, which can often be more than half (60%) experiencing burnout.

7. Hobby Development

Burned-out healthcare workers have little energy to take care of themselves with proper nourishment, exercise, and sleep , let alone ensure they have hobbies and social activities. It is incumbent on each person to begin to carve out time to make each day, both inside and outside of work, memorable.

Many people feel like they can just set aside time to do the things they like most during their retirement. On the contrary, take all your interests and nurture them throughout your life. A hobby is not only what helps one achieve satisfaction right now but also provides a greater sense of resilience. Studies support that taking these steps to develop leisure activities can strengthen one's health and well-being.

I can say that music has truly helped me manage stress and develop creative skills. The opportunity to play the guitar was an unexpected gift during my medical school years. One of my favorite third-year medical rotations was my month in The Gambia, West Africa. After the long days in the clinic, the evenings turned into an elective course in music. My physician mentor brought her guitar. When the village's electricity shut off every evening, playing the guitar was an excellent way to pass the time under the glow of candlelight. We also attended evening concerts at a music camp organized by a Norwegian musician who hosted musicians from all over West Africa. From that time on, music has provided me with relaxation, entertainment, and a chance for continued learning.

Learning new skills allows you to get out of your comfort zone, enriching your life in return. You might wonder how to find time to learn something else during medical school. Time spent away from studying can provide a student an outlet for basic needs and personal growth. My advice to the reader is to schedule at least an hour each day to learn something new. You could do something like attend a foreign language meet-up group for an hour a week or attend skill-building workshops, such as woodworking, art, writing, and other crafts. There are smartphone meeting apps that make planning almost effortless.

Strategies to Develop Resilience to Burnout

1. Workload Reduction and Increased Autonomy

2. Mindfulness Practices

3. Shared Dialogues and Social Support

4. Volunteerism and International Humanitarian Work

5. Mentorship

6. Non-Clinical Practices

7. Hobby Development

Summary: Resilience is Possible

Burnout is long-term stress that can manifest as emotional fatigue, depersonalization, and a lost sense of fulfillment. Physicians can develop skills to protect themselves from burnout and serve as stewards in supporting others. The goal is to equip oneself with resilience and enhance their care to create a more fulfilling experience. Tomorrow's doctors can incorporate these strategies early on and develop behaviors to withstand compromising health for professional expectations.

Administrative and education committees also need to be aware of and include resilience programs that address burnout for their workforce. Commensality dinners and mindfulness seminars may be helpful initiatives from these groups. It is essential to frame burnout as a joint endeavor between physicians, practice members, and administrators.

CHAPTER 11

Closing Remarks

Learning is the only thing the mind never exhausts,
never fears, and never regrets.
Leonardo Da Vinci

Medicines cure diseases,
but only doctors can cure patients.
Carl Jung

The doctor of the future will give no medicine but will instruct his patient in the care of the human frame in diet and in the cause and prevention of disease.
Thomas Edison

To find health should be the object of the doctor.
Anyone can find disease.
Andrew Taylor Still

Medical school is an exhilarating educational experience, but it is only the beginning. There are so many opportunities and life lessons that a career in medicine brings to the receptive and curious doctor. It bestows on the practitioner a window into addressing an individual's life challenges, fears, and uncertainties. Therein lies the solution to finding health. There is no privilege more significant than being entrusted with this responsibility.

A Physician is a Lifelong Teacher and Learner

Within the Hippocratic and Osteopathic Oaths are profound statements about the importance of teaching. A mentor shares a place of esteem equivalent to a student's parents. And later, students become teachers, passing on their knowledge to subsequent generations. However, in contradistinction to teaching children, physicians function as facilitators to medical students, interns, and residents (Cheesman, 2009). Skilled mentors can guide trainees to invigorating learning moments when a clinical context galvanizes book information. As I recall the most instrumental rotations in my development, the mentors were the reason.

Patient care gives a context, attaching facts to a purpose. From the first half of medical school to the second half, education transforms from book to applied knowledge. Students develop reasoning skills for an improved decision-making framework along with foundational knowledge. When physicians meet diagnostic uncertainty, their training equips them with ways to address it. The most common cause of errors stems from bias, and doctors may miss what their thinking does not consider. However, active listening and skilled decision-making can still bring a physician toward the next steps in a workup.

A physician is a life-long learner. Every clinic day brings the opportunity for a new lesson and "first." I recently saw a patient with elevated liver tests and other studies suggesting he had autoimmune hepatitis (AIH). A work-up for infectious causes was negative. I reviewed articles on the condition and how to distinguish it from other diseases and ordered follow-up blood tests. As his status worsened, I transferred him to the hospital to have a diagnostic liver biopsy, receive a consultation with a hepatologist, and begin treatment (initially prednisone). He was the first patient I saw with AIH in my career. I was pleased to see him return feeling better and on the road to recovery.

After passing medical licensing and board certification examinations, most state licensing boards require at least 40 hours of continuing medical education (CME) every two years to maintain active status. Physicians may attend conferences or obtain the credits online. They may pursue specific training areas or seek to strengthen their general knowledge base. Meetings engender a sense of community and a way to disseminate novel thinking and research. Physicians return recharged and can apply their new knowledge immediately to their practice.

Mostly, Patients Heal Themselves

The doctor-patient relationship is a privilege, not an assumption. Doctors can have a tremendous role in addressing the link between their patients' chronic diseases and behaviors within a safe and nurturing context. A Carl Jung quote reads, "medicines can cure diseases, but only doctors can cure patients." However, the use of "cure" in this statement is misleading. Most medicines only treat the symptoms that surface while an underlying disease progresses. They do not act directly on the causes. Additionally, doctors can offer their insight, compassionate listening, and counseling, but they do not cure patients.

Patients must cure themselves of chronic diseases. But seldom would they be successful alone. As the ACE study suggests, disease results from an adaptation to trauma (Felitti, 1998). Healing begins as individuals adjust their behavioral patterns and release the trauma's hold. As the constructs are subconscious and deeply rooted, doctors and their clinical teams can partner with patients as navigators, teachers, and coaches. Support groups can also increase accountability and motivation. As Malcolm X said, "when i is replaced with we, even illness becomes wellness." Tomorrow's doctors serve in the collaborative effort to support a patient's wellness journey.

Pre-medical Fears

Pre-medical students often wonder whether becoming a physician is worth the years and loans needed for training[68]. I certainly did when I was considering medical school. It is essential to explore the source of any doubt. It could stem from ambivalence to medicine as a career; the doubt could be a fear, such as losing flexibility, a costly commitment, or the pressure of academic rigor.

My advice for uncertainty would be to shadow physicians. A study of premedical students showed a significant improvement in student awareness of physician duties and patient care following a shadowing program (Wang, 2015). The pandemic led to a halt in observer opportunities, but online shadowing sites have filled the gaps. These opportunities provide first-hand observation and a chance to learn about a physician's unique professional journey. The endpoint is the insight to decide whether to apply for medical school or not.

As for the fear, medical school is a commitment that is not for everyone. But it is worth it if you are feeling a calling. It has become more common and acceptable to take a gap year before applying for or entering medical school. Traditional college-age students seldom have opportunities to gain life experience outside of the educational context. The extra time can allow a student a chance to volunteer locally or internationally, research, travel, or do health-related work (e.g., scribing in a clinic). Sometimes a year can be enough time for someone to indulge in their curiosities and start medical school rejuvenated.

My concerns as a pre-medical student were the time commitment and the rigorous coursework. After college graduation, I packed a backpack and boarded a plane to England to begin a two-month trip through Europe with two of my friends. Although the thought of extending the trip for a year occurred as I was preparing to return, it was long enough to satisfy my craving for an adventure. When I began medical school, I approached the assignments with a genuine interest that allayed my fears of the challenges, albeit the curiosity did not reduce my study time.

"Full-filling" a Career and the Parable of the Stonecutter

It is hard to believe that I have spent more than half of my life as a doctor. Students often ask me whether I would become a doctor again if I could go back in time. The answer is a resounding "Yes!"

My career is a gift. My cup is overflowing. This profession has taken me around the world to places like Africa, South America, and various parts of the United States. I have worked in practice settings like clinics, hospitals, departments of public health, academic centers, and even a prison. There is flexibility in how I can arrange my schedule, and I leave one day a week for creative time. My income is substantial, even though it is the physician average.

I conclude with the Taoist parable of the stonecutter (Ward, 2020). The story begins with a lowly stonecutter using his tools to break off stone pieces from a mountain. The stonecutter takes a journey of discovery fueled by the desire to become increasingly more powerful. He is transformed into a lord and then natural forces like the sun, the clouds, and the wind. He becomes the clouds when he observes them blocking the sun. But upon discovering how the wind moves them effortlessly, he changes into the wind. He wields tremendous power as the wind but realizes that mountains stand unaffected. After the man transforms into a mountain, he hears a stonecutter chipping away at his base.

The parable tells us that power lies within all of us, no matter what we do in life. There will always seem to be something that appears better, but it turns out to be less than was desired. Rather than living a life dictated by desire, the parable reminds us that every moment along the way is important. Becoming a doctor or any profession is not a destination but part of a transformation. Each day is a journey of developing skills, understanding ways we can contribute to the betterment of others, and appreciating the moment's happiness. That is at the heart of fulfillment.

Best wishes on your journey!

References

Chapter 1: On Becoming a Physicial: My Journey

AACOM website. US Colleges of Osteopathic Medicine. www.aacom.org.

AAMC website. Medical School Enrollment More Diverse in 2021. www.aamc.org.

AAMC website. Core Competencies for Entering Medical Students. www.aamc.org/services/admissions-lifecycle/competencies-entering-medical-students

AOA website. 2020-21 report tracks increased growth in the osteopathic profession. AOA website: https://osteopathic.org/about/aoa-statistics/.

Barré-Sinoussi, et al. Isolation of a T-lymphotropic retrovirus from a patient at risk for Acquired Immunedeficiency Syndrome (AIDS). Science. 1983; 220(4599):868-71. doi: 10.1126/science.6189183.

Desy J, Coderre S, Veale P, Busche K, Woloschuk W, McLaughlin K. Can we predict failure in licensure exams from medical students' undergraduate academic performance? Can Med Educ J. 2021;

12(6): 6-13. Doi: 10.36834/cmej.68172.

Dudley J, McLaughlin S, Lee T. Why So Many Women Physicians are Quitting. Harvard Business Review. Jan 19, 2022. https://hbr.org/2022 01/why-so-many-women-physicians-are-quitting.

Gallo R, Montagnier L. The Discovery of HIV as the Cause of AIDS. N Engl J Med. 2003. 349:2283-2285.

Kerr E. 10 Med Schools with the Lowest Acceptance Rates. US News. April 13, 2021. www.usnews.com/education/best-graduate-school/the-short-list-grad-school/articles/medical.

Koh G, Khoo H, Wong M, Koh D. The effects of problem-based learning during medical school on physician competency: a systematic review. CMAJ. 2008; 178(1):34-41.

Ly D, Seabury S, Jena A, Newhouse R. Differences in incomes of physicians in the United States by race and sex: observational study. BMJ. 2016; 353: i2923. doi: 10.1136/bmj.i2923.

Michas F. Total active physicians in the US 2021, by state. www.statista.com/statistics/186269/total-active-physicians-in-the-us.

Tan S Y, Zia J K. Andrew Taylor Still (1828-1917): founder of osteopathic medicine. Singapore Med J. 2007; 48(11): 975.

Tyrone, D, Paolucii E, Violato C. The Predictive Validity of the MCAT for Medical School Performance and Medical Board Licensing Examinations: A Meta-Analysis of the Published Research. Academic Medicine. 2007; 82(1): 100-106. doi:10/1097/01.ACM.0000249787.25186.b7.

Vaillant G. et al. Some Psychologic Vulnerabilities of Physicians. N Engl J Med. 1972; 287:372-375.

Chapter 2: The Evolution of the Modern Health Paradigm

Anderson G, Horvath J. The Growing Burden of Chronic Disease in America. Public Health Reports. 2004; Vol 119.

Andraska E, Alabi O, Dorsey C, Erben Y, Velazquez G, Franco-Mesa C, Sachdez U. Health care disparities during the COVID-19 pandemic. Semin Vasc Surg. 2021; 34(3): 82-88.

Blakemore E. Why plague doctors wore those strange beaked masks. National Geographic. March 12, 2020.

Borrell-Carrió F, Suchman A, Epstein R. The Biopsychosocial Model 25 Years Later: Principles, Practice, and Scientific Inquiry. Ann Fam Med. 2004; 2(6): 576-582.

Butler T. Plague history: Yersin's discovery of the causative bacterium in 1894 enabled, in the subsequent century, scientific progress in understanding the disease and development of treatments and vaccines. Clin Microbiol Infect. 2014; 20(3): 202-9. doi: 10.1111/1469-0691.12530.

Cleeremans A, Achouui D, et al. Learning to Be Conscious. Trends in Cognitive Sciences. 2020; Vol 24(2): 112-123.

Dearing J, Cox J. Diffusion of Innovations Theory, Principles, and Practice. Health Affairs. 2018; 37(2):183-190.

Dunn PM. Galen (AD 129-200) of Pergamon: anat

omist and experimental physiologist. Arch Dis Child Fetal Neonatal Ed. 2003; 88:F441-F443.

Engel G. The need for a new medical model: a challenge for biomedicine. Science. 1977; 196(4286): 129-36. doi: 10.1126/science.847460.

FDA. COVID-19 Vaccines. www.fda.gov/ emergency-preparedness-and-response/coronavirus-disease-2019-covid-19/covid-19-vaccines

Felitti V, et al. Relationship of Childhood Abuse and Household Dysfunction to Many of the Leading Causes of Death in Adults. The Adverse Childhood Experiences (ACE) Study. Am J of Prev Med. 1998; Vol 14(4):245-382.

Flaskerud J. Temperament and Personality: From Galen to DSM. Issues in Mental Health Nursing. 2012; 33:631-634. doi: 10.3109/01612840.2011.647256.

Glatter K, Finkelman. History of the Plague: An Ancient Pandemic for the Age of COVID-19. Am J Med. 2021; 132(2): 176-181. doi: 10.1016/j.amjmed.2020.08.019.

Green L, Mehr D. What alters physicians' decisions to admit to the coronary care unit? Journal Fam Practice. 1997; 45(3): 219-226.

Greenhalgh T. Miasmas, mental models, and preventive public health: some philosophical reflections on science in the COVID-19 pandemic. Interface Focus. 2021; 11(6):20210017. doi: 10.1098/rsfs.2021.0017.

Heikkinen E. A paradigm shift: from disease to health orientation. The Aging Male. 2000; 3: 171-176.

Heldreth T. Avicenna's Canon of Medicine: Influences and Implications. A Thesis Submitted to the Faculty of Baylor University. Baylor-ir.tdl.org.

Johnson S. The ghost map: a street, an epidemic, and the hidden power of urban networks. 2008. London, UK: Penguin.

Kannadan A. History of the Miasma Theory of Disease. ESAAI. 2018; Vol 16(18). https://dc.cod.edu/essai/vol16/iss1/18.

Kotchoubey B. Human Consciousness: Where is it from and What is it for. Front Psych. 2018; 9: 567. doi: 10.3389/fpsyg.2018.00567.

Kuhn, T. The Structure of Scientific Revolutions. 1962. Intl Encyclopedia of Unified Science.

Lamme V. Can neuroscience reveal the true nature of consciousness? Source: www.nyu.edu/gsas/dept/philo/courses/consciousness05/LammeNeuroscience.pdf

Lagay F. The Legacy of Humoral Medicine. Virtual Mentor. 2002; 4(7). doi: 10.1001/virtualmentor.2002.4.7.mhst1-0207.

McCulloch M, et al. Diagnostic Accuracy of Canine Scent Detection in Early- and Late-Stage Lung and Breast Cancers. Integrative Cancer Therapies. 2006.

Patel JA. Poverty, inequality, and COVID-19: the forgotten vulnerable. Public Health. 2020; 183: 110-111.

Poppick, L. Let us now Praise the Invention of the Microscope. Smithsonian Magazine.
March 30, 2017.

Raghupathi W, and Raghupathi V. An Empirical Study of Chronic Diseases in the United States:
A Visual Analytics Approach to Public Health. Int J. Environ Res Public Health. 2018; 15(3): 431.

Roberts S, Chandler G, and Kalmakis K. A model for trauma-informed primary care. J Am Assoc of Nurse Practitioners. 2019; 31(2): 139-144.

Schroeder SA. We can do better— Improving the health of the American people. N Engl J Med.
2007; 357: 1221-1228.

Wade D. Do biomedical models of illness make for good healthcare systems? BMJ. 2004; 329(7479): 1398-1401. doi:10.1136/bmj/329.7479.1398

West J. Galen and the beginnings of Western physiology. Am Journ Phys Lung Cellular and Molecular Phys. 2014: pp1-16. doi.org/10.1152/ajplung.00123.2014.

West R, Russell M, Stanovich K. Cognitive sophistication does not attenuate the bias blind spot. Journal of Personality and Social Psychology. 2012; 103(3): 506-519. doi: org/10.1037/a0028857.

WHO Coronavirus (COVID-19) Dashboard | WHO Coronavirus (COVID-19) Dashboard with Vaccination Data. https://covid19.who.int.

Yaribeygi H, Panahi Y, Sahraei H, Johnston T, Sehebkar A. The impact of stress on body function: A review. EXCLI J. 2017; 16: 1057-1072.

Chapter 3: Transcending Bias in Clinical Diagnosis

Barnett M, Boddupalli D, Nundy S. Comparative Accuracy of Diagnosis by Collective Intelligence of Multiple Physicians vs. Individual Physicians. JAMA Netw Open. 2019; 2(3):e190096. doi: 10/1001/jamanetworkopen.2019.0096.

Bhamidipati A. Pulmonary embolism: Why we miss it, and how do we get better? Emdocs online. https:// laptrinhx.com/news/ pulmonary-embolism-why-do-we-miss-it-and-how-do-we-get-better-mazxmRb/

Ceresoli M, Lo Bianco G, Gianotti L, Nespoli L. Inflammation management in acute diverticulitis: current perspectives. J Inflamm Res. 2018; 11: 239-246. doi: 10.2147/JIR.S142990.

Croskerry P. Achieving Quality in Clinical Decision Making: Cognitive Strategies and Detection of Bias. Academic Emergency Med. 2002; 9: 1183-1204.

Croskery P. The importance of cognitive errors in diagnosis and strategies to minimize them. Acad Med. 2003; 78(8): 775-780.

Croskerry P, Signhal G, Mamede S. Cognitive debiasing 1: origins of bias and theory of debiasing. BMJ Qual Saf. 2013; 22(Suppl 2): ii58-64. doi: 10.1136/bmjqs-2012-001712.

Densen P. Challenges and Opportunities Facing Medical Education. Trans Am Clin Climatol Assoc. 2011; 122: 45-58.

Elston D. Confirmation bias in medical decision-making. Journ Am Academy Derm. 2019. Vol 82 (3): 572. doi: https://doi.org/10.1016/j.jaad.2019.06.1286.

Ely J, Graber M, Croskerry P. Checklists to reduce diagnostic errors. Acad Med. 2011; 86(3): 307-13. doi: 10.1097/ACM.0b13e31820824cd.

Federation of State Medical Boards. Assessing Scope of Practice in Health Care Delivery: Critical Questions in Assuring Public Access and Safety. 2005. www.fmsb.org/siteassets.advocacy/policies/assessing-scope-in-practice.

Graber M, Franklin N, Gordon R. Diagnostic error in internal medicine. Arch Intern Med. 2005; 165(13): 1493-9.

Hampton JR, Harrison MJ, Mitchell JR, Prichard JS, Seymour C. Relative contributions of history-taking, physical exam, and lab investigation to diagnosis and management of medical outpatients. Br Med J. 1975; 2(5969):486-489.

Helwig J. 1964 May, The Reader's Digest, Vol 84, My Most Unforgettable Character. Pg. 129.

Herschberger PJ, et al. Understanding and addressing cognitive bias in medical education. Adv Health Sci Educ Theory Pract. 1996; 1(2):221-6. doi: 10.1007/BF00162919.

Kahneman D. (2011). Thinking, Fast and Slow. New York. Farrar, Straus, and Giroux.

Kim H, Hong H, Yoon SH. Diagnostic Performance of CT, and Reverse Transcriptase Polymerase Chain Reaction for Coronavirus Disease 2019: A Meta-Analysis. Radiology. 2020; 296: E145-E155.

Kruger J, Dunning D. Unskilled and unaware of it: how difficulties in recognizing one's own incompetence lead to inflated self-assessments. J Pers Soc Psychol. 1999; 77(6): 1121-34. doi: 10.1037//0022-3514.77.6.1121.

Langford B, Daneman N, Leung V, Langford D. Cognitive bias: how understanding its impact on antibiotic prescribing decisions can help advance antimicrobial stewardship. JAC-Antimicrobial Resistance. 2020; 2(4). doi.org/10.1093/jacamr/dlaa107.

Lakoff G, Johnson M. (1999). Philosophy in the flesh: the embodied mind and its challenge to Western thought. New York: Basic Books.

Laws MB, Lee Y, Taubin, T, Rogers W, Wilson I. Factors associated with patient recall of key information in ambulatory specialty care visits: Results of an innovative methodology. PloS ONE. 2018; 13(2): e0191940. https://doi.org/10.1371/journal.pone.0191940.

Marewski J, Gigerenzer G. Heuristic decision making in medicine. Dialogues Clin Neurosci. 2012; 14(1):77-89.

Motta M, Callaghan T, Sylvester S. Knowing less but presuming more: Dunning-Kruger effects and the endorsement of anti-vaccine policy attitudes. Soc Sci Med. 2018; 211: 274-281. doi: 10.1016/j.socscimed.2018.06.032. Epub 2018 Jun 25.

Nichols LO, Mirvis DM. Physician-patient communication: does it matter? Tenn Med. 1998; 91(3):94-6.

Olson K. "Oh, by the Way…": Agenda Setting in Office Visits. FPM. 2002; 9(10):63-64.

Pullan S, Dey M. Vaccine hesitancy and anti-vaccination in the time of COVID-19: A Google Trend analysis. Vaccine. 2021; 39(14): 1877-1881. doi: 10.1016/j.vaccine.2021.03.019.

Rounds PG. Anchoring bias with critical implications. Aorn J. 2016;103:658-631.

Semigran H, Linder JA, Gidengil C, Mehrotra A. Evaluation of symptoms checkers for self-diagnosis and triage: audit study. BMJ. 2015; 351:h3480.

Semigran H, Levine D, Nundy S, et al. Comparison of Physician and Computer Diagnostic Accuracy. JAMA Internal Medicine. 2016; 176(12): 1860-1861. doi:10:1001/jamainternmed.2016.6001.

Shi H, Han X, Jiang N, Cao Y, Alwalid O, Gu J, Fan Y, Zheng C. Radiological findings from 81 patients with COVID-19 pneumonia in Wuhan, China: a descriptive study. Lancet Infect Dis. 2020; 20(4):425-434.

Sladek R, Phillips P, Bond M. Measurement properties of the Inventory of Cognitive Bias in Medicine (ICBM). BMC Med Inform Decis Mak. 2008; 8:20. Doi: 10/1186/1472-6947-8-20.

Stanovich K, West R. Individual differences in reasoning: Implications for the rationality debate? Behavioral and Brain Sciences. 2000; 23: 645-726.

Stiegler M, Tung A. Cognitive Processes in Anesthesiology Decision Making. Anesthesiology. 2014; Vol 120: 204-217.

Swee-Lin Tan S, Goonawardene N. Internet Health Seeking and the Patient-Physician Relationship: A Systematic Review. J Med Internet Res. 2017; 19(1): e9. doi: 10.2196/jmir.5729.

Wang Y, Dong C, Hu Y, Li C, Ren Q, Zhang X, Shi H, Zhou M. Temporal Changes of CT Findings in 90 Patients with COVID-19 Pneumonia: A Longitudinal Study.

Chapter 4: On Medical Errors

Aaronson E, Quinn G, Wong C, Murray AM, Carter P, Einbinder J, Schiff G. Missed diagnosis of cancer in primary care: Insights from malpractice claims data. Journ Healthcare Risk Management. 2019; Vol 39(2): 19-29.

Brady A. Error and discrepancy in radiology: inevitable or avoidable? Insights Imaging. 2017; 8(1): 171-182. doi: 10.1007/s13244-016-0534-1.

CRICO/RMF. 2010. Protecting providers. Promoting safety. www.rmf.harvard.edu/high-risk-areas/diagnosis/index.aspx.

Gong J, et al. Metastasis in renal cell carcinoma: Biology and implications for therapy. Asian J Urol. 2016; 3(4): 286-292. doi: 10.1016/j.ajur.2016.08.006.

Johnson TJ, Hickey RW, Switzer GE, Miller E, Winger DG, Nguyen M, et al. The Impact of Cognitive Stressors in the Emergency Department on Physical Implicit Racial Bias. Academic Emergency Medicine. 2016; 13 Jan. Vol 23, Issue 3.

Leape L, et al. The nature of adverse events in hospitalized patients. Results of the Harvard Medical Practice Study II. N Engl J Med. 1991; 324: 37-84.

Markarey M, Daniel M. Medical error— the third leading cause of death in the US. BMJ. 2016; 353:i2139. doi: https://doi.org/10.1136/bmj.i2139.

Mewara A, Goyal K, Sehgal R. Neurocysticercosis: A disease of neglect. Trop Parasitol. 2013; 3(2): 106-113. doi: 10.4103/2229-57070.12211.

Neale G, Hogan H, Sevdalis N. Misdiagnosis: analysis based on case record review with proposals aimed to improve diagnostic processes. Clin Med (Lond). 2011; 11(4): 317-21. doi: 10.7861/clinmdicine.11-4-317.

Rodziewicz T, Houseman B, Hipskind J. Medical Error Reduction and Prevention. (2022).

StatPearls [Internet]. StatPearls Publishing: Treasure Island, Florida. Sullivan E, Schofield SJ. Cognitive bias in clinical medicine. J R Coll Physicians Edinb. 2018; 48: 225-232. doi: 10.4997/JRCPE.2018.306

Singh H, Giardina TD, Meyer A, et al. Types and origins of diagnostic errors in primary care settings. JAMA Intern Med. 2013; 173: 418-25.

Tiwary et al. Poor communication by health care professionals may lead to life-threateningcomplications: examples from two case reports. Wellcome Open Res. 2019; 4: 7.

Tudor G, Finlay D, Taub N. An assessment of inter-observer agreement and accuracy when reporting plain radiographs. Clinical Radiology. 1997; Vol 52(3): 235-238.

Zejnullahu Valon, Bicaj B, Zejnullahu Vjosa, Hamza A. Retained Surgical Foreign Bodies After Surgery. Mac Journ Medical Sciences. 2017; 5(1):97-100.

Schantz P, et al. Neurocystercosis in an Orthodox Jewish Community in New York City. N Engl J Med. 1992; 327: 692-695. doi: 10.1056/NEJM199209033271004

Chapter 5: The Generalist and the Specialist

Ashton H. The diagnosis and management of benzodiazepine dependence. Curr Opin Psychiatry. 2005; Vol 18:249-255.

Association of American Medical Colleges. 2016 Physician Specialty Data Book. November 2014.

Association of American Medical Colleges. The Complexities of Physician Supply and Demand Projections from 2018 to 2033. June 2016. Aamc.org/media/45976/download.

Canadian Institute for Health Information. Drug use among seniors in Canada, 2016. Ottawa, Ontario. http://www.cihi.ca/sites/default/files/document/drug-use-among-seniors-2016-en-web.pdf.

Donohoe M. Comparing Generalist and Specialty Care. Discrepancies, Deficiencies, and Excesses. Archives Intern Med. 1998; Vol 158.

Golchin N, Frank S, Vince A, Isham L, Meropol S. Polypharmacy in the elderly. J Res Pharm Pract. 2015; 4(2): 85-88.

IDSA. Career Paths in ID. www.idsociety org/professional-development/education--training/career-paths-in-id/

Johnson J, Bootman J. Drug-related morbidity and mortality. A cost-of-illness model. Arch Intern Med. 1995; 155(18): 1949-56.

Landon B, et al. Physician specialization and the quality of care for human immunodeficiency virus infection. Arch Intern Med. 2005; 165(10): 1133-9.

Leipzig RM, Cumming RG, Tinetti ME. Drugs and falls in order people: a systematic review and meta-analysis: II. Cardiac and analgesic drugs. J Am Geriatr Soc. 1999; 47(1): 40-50.

Medscape. Physician Compensation Report 2018. www.medscape.com/sites/public/physicain-comp/2018.

Medscape. Medscape Lifestyle Report 2017: Race and Ethnicity, Bias, and Burnout. www.medscape.com/features/slideshow/lifestyle/2017/overview#pages=2.

Rosenblatt R, Hart G. Physicians and rural America. West J Med. 2000; 173(5): 348-351. doi: 10.1136/ewjm.173.5.348.

Starfield B, Shi L, Macinko J. Contribution of Primary Care to Health Systems and Health. Milbank Q. 2005; 83(3): 457-502.

Safai Y. Popular anti-anxiety medications may be highly addictive, FDA says. But is this warning too late? ABC News. https://abcnews.go.com/health/popular-anti-anxiety-medication.

Scott I, Hilmer S, Reeve E, Potter K, Le Couteur D, Rigby D, et al. Reducing inappropriate polypharmacy: the process of describing. JAMA Intern Med. 2015; 175(5): 827-34.

Wagner S, Mehta A, Laber D. Rituximab-induced interstitial lung disease. Am J Hematol. 2007; 82:916-919.

Zed P, Abu-Laban R, Balen R, Loewen P, Hohl C, Brubacher J, Wilbur K, Wiens M, Samoy L, Lascaria K, Purssell R. Incidence, severity, and preventability of medication-related visits to the emergency department: a prospective study. CMAJ. 2008; 178(12): 1563-1569.

Chapter 6: On the Difficult Diagnosis and Sudden Changes in Health

Aiarzaguena J, et al. The diagnostic challenges presented by patients with medically unexplained symptoms in general practice. Scand J Prim Health Care. 2008; 26(2): 99-105. doi: 10.1080/02813430802048662.

Bonanno F. Physiopathology of shock. J Emerg Trauma Shock. 2011; 3(2) 222-232.

Cerny T, Borisch B, Introna M, Johnson P, Rose A. Mechanism of action of rituximab. Anticancer Drugs. 2002; 13 Suppl 2: S3-10.

Cirino C, et al. Transfusion-Associated Babesiosis with an Atypical Time Course after Nonmyeloablative Transplantation for Sickle Cell Disease. Ann Intern Med. 2008; 148(10): 794-795

Debi U, Ravisankar V, Prasad K, Sinha S, Sharma A. Abdominal tuberculosis of the gastrointestinal tract: Revisited. World J Gastroenterol. 2014; 20(40): 14831-148540. doi: 10.3748/wpj.v20.i40.14831.

Donner-Banzhoff N. Solving the Diagnostic Challenge: A Patient-Centered Approach. Annals of Family Medicine. 2018; Vol 16(4).

Ebner D, Kisiel J. Stool-Based tests for Colorectal Cancer Screening: Performance Benchmarks Lead to High Expected Efficacy. Curr Gastroenterol Rep. 2020; 22(7): 32. doi: 10.1007/s11894-020-00770-6.

Engdahl J, Bang A, Lindqvist J, Herlitz J. Can we define patients with no and those with some chance of survival when found in asystole out of hospital? Am J Cardiol. 2000; 86(6): 610-4. doi: 10.1016/s0002-9149(00)01037-7.

Tawil SE, Muir KW. Thrombolysis and thrombectomy for acute ischaemic stroke. Clin Med. 2017 Apr;17(2):161-165. doi: 10.7861/clinmedicine.17-2-161. PMID: 28365630; PMCID: PMC6297620.

Griffin G, Shenoi S, Hughes G. Hemophagocytic lymphohistiocytosis: An update on pathogenesis, diagnosis, and therapy. Best Pract Res Clin Rheumatol. 2020; 34(4):101515. doi: 10.1016/j.berh.2020.101515. Epub 2020 May 7.

Gu W et al. 2019. Clinical Metagenomic Next-Generation Sequencing for Pathogen Detection. Annu Rev Pathol. 2019; Jan 24:14:319-338.

Hurt C, Tammaro D. Diagnostic Evaluation of Mononucleosis-Like Illnesses. Am J Med. 2007; Vol 120(10): 911.E1-911.E8. doi.org/10.1016.j.amjmed.2006.12.011.

Ladabaum U, et al. Colorectal Cancer Screening with Blood-Based Biomarkers: Cost-Effectiveness of Methylated Septin 9 DNA versus Current Strategies. Cancer Epidemiol Biomarkers Prev. 2013; 22(9): 1567-76. doi: 10.1158/1055-9965.EPI-13-0204.

Lecuit M and M Eliot. The diagnosis of infectious diseases by whole genome next generation sequencing: a new era is opening. Front Cell Infect Microbiol. 2014; 4: 25. doi:10.3389/fcimb.2014.00025.

Levin A, Krause P. Transfusion-transmitted babesiosis: Is it time to screen the blood supply? Curr Opin Hematol. 2016; Nov; 23(6): 573-580.

Lyratzopoulos G, Wadle J, Rubin G. Rethinking diagnostic delay in cancer: how difficult is the diagnosis? BMJ. 2014; 349:g7400. doi:10.1136/bmj.g7400.

Patel T, Karle E, Krvavac A. Avoiding Unnecessary Repeat Laboratory Testing. Cureus. 2019; 11(10): e5872. doi: 10.7759/cureus.5872.

Sarkar U. Challenges of Making a Diagnosis in the Outpatient Setting: A Multi-Site Survey of Primary Care Physicians. BMJ Qual Saf. 2012; 21(8): 641-648.

Saghafinia M, Motamedi M, et al. Survival after in-hospital cardiopulmonary resuscitation in a major referral center. Saudi J Anaesth. 2010; 4(2): 68-71.

Saver JL. Time is Brain – Quantified. Stroke. 2006; 37:263-266.

Shute D. 2019. Coping with grief: How physicians can heal after patient death. Website: www.physicianpractice.com/view/coping-grief-how-physicians-can-heal-after-patient-deaths.

Terhune C. 2017. The $200 billion perils of unnecessary medical tests. PBS news hour. www.pbs.org.

Chapter 7: The Difficult Encounter

Alozai U, McPherson P. Malingering. StatPearls [Internet]. Treasure Island (FL). StatPearls Publishing. Accessed 7/21/2022.

CDC. Drug Overdose Deaths in the U.S. Top 100,000 Annually. 2021. www.cdc.gov/pressreleases/2021/20211117.html

CDC. Prescription Opioid Overdose Death Maps. Drug Overdose. CDC Injury Center.
www.cdc.gov/drugoverdose/deaths/prescription/maps.html?msclkid=37e670f9c13c11ec9266afc2c33d426e

Chang H, Daubresse M, Kruszewski S, Alexander G. Prevalence and treatment of pain in EDs in the United States, 2000 to 2010. Am J Emergency Med. 2014; Vol 32(5): 421-431.

D'Souza R, Lang M, Eldrige J. (2022). Prescription Drug Monitoring Program. StatPearls
[Internet]. StatPearls Publishing. Treasure Island (FL).

Evans C, Cahill C. Neurobiology of opioid dependence in creating addiction vulnerability.
F1000Res. 2016; 5:F1000 Faculty Rev01748.
doi: 10.12688/f1000research.8369.1.eCollection 2016.

Gatchel R, et al. The biopsychosocial approach to chronic pain: Scientific advances and future
directions. Psychological Bulletin. 2007; 133(4): 581-624.
doi: 10.1037/0033-2909.133.4.581.

Interagency Pain Research Coordinating Committee. National Pain Strategy: A Comprehensive Population Health-Level Strategy for Pain. US Department of Health and Human Services, National Institutes of Health; 2016.

Kosten T, George T. The neurobiology of opioid dependence: implications for treatment. Sci Pract Perspect. 2002; 1(1): 13-20. doi: 10.1151/spp021113.

National Institute on Drug Abuse (NIDA). Overdose Death Rates. https://nida.nih.gov/drug-topics/trends-statistics/overdose-death-rates

Palmieri J, Stern T. Lies in the Doctor-Patient Relationship. Prim Care Companion J Clin Psychiatry. 2009; 11(4): 163-168. doi: 10.4088/PCC.09r00780.

Portenoy R, Foley K. Chronic use of opioid analgesics in non-malignant pain: report of 38 cases. Pain. 1986; 25(2): 171-186. doi: 10.1016/0304-3959(86)90091-6.

Rayner L, Hotopf M, et al. Depression in patients with chronic pain attending a specialized pain treatment centre: prevalence and impact on health care costs. Pain. 2016; 157(7): 1472-9. doi: 10.1097/j.pain.0000000000000542.

Sokol R, Pines R, Chew A. Multidisciplinary Approach for Managing Complex Pain and Addiction in Primary Care: A Qualitative Study. Ann Fam Med. 2021; 19(3): 224-231. doi: 10.1370/afm.2648.

Strickler G, Zhang K, Halpin J, Bohnert A, Baldwin G, Kreiner P. Effects of mandatory prescription drug monitoring program (PDMP) use laws on prescriber registration and use and on risky prescribing. Drug and Alcohol Dependence. 2019; Vol 199: 1-9. doi.org/10.1016/j.drugalcdep.2019.02.010.

US Department of Health and Human Services. Opioid Crisis Statistics.
Website: www.hhs.gov/opioids/about-the-epidemic/opioid-crisis-statistics/index.html

Chapter 8: The Power of Listening, Communication, and Collaboration

Beckman HB, Frankel RM. The effect of physician behavior on the collection of data. Ann Intern Med. 1984; 101:692-5.

Biglu M, Nateq F, Ghohazadeh M, Asghardzadeh A. Communication Skills of Physicians and Patients' Satisfaction. Mater Sociomed. 2017; Sept; 29(3):192-195.

Dang B, et al. Building trust and rapport early in the new doctor-patient relationship: a longitudinal qualitative study. BMC Medical Education. 2017; 17 (32). https://doi.org/10.1186/s12909-017-0868-5.

D'Amour D, Ferrada-Videla M, Rodriguez L, Beaulieu M. The Conceptual Basis for Interprofessional Collaboration: Core Concepts and Theoretical Frameworks. Journ Interprofess Care. 2005; 19116-131.

Dyche L, Swiderski D. The Effect of Physician Solicitation Approaches on Ability to Identify Patient Concerns. J Gen Intern Med. 2005; 20(3):267-270.

Gaspari R, Dayno M, Briones J, Blehar D. Comparison of computerized tomography and ultrasound in diagnosing soft tissue abscesses. Critical Ultrasound Journal. 2012; 4: 5

Goldman L. Hospitalists as a cure for hospitalism. Trans Am Clin Climatol Assoc. 2003; 114: 37-50. PMID: 12813910.

International Listening Association; 2009. www.listen.org

Jagosh J, Boudreau JD, Steinert Y, MacDonald ME, Ingram L. The importance of physician listening from the patients' perspective: Enhancing diagnosis, healing, and the doctor-patient relationship. Patient Education and Counseling. 2011; 85: 369-374.

King A, Hoppe R. Best Practice for Patient-Centered Communication: A Narrative Review. Journal of Grad Med Education. 2013; 5(3): 385-393. doi: 10.4300/JGME-D-13-00072.1.

Koenig T, et al. Core personal competencies important to entering students' success in medical school: what are they and how could they be assessed early in the admission process? Acad Med. 2013; 88(5):603-13. Doi: 10.1097/ACM.ob013e31828b3389.

Morley L, Cashell A. Collaboration in Health Care. J Med Imaging Rad Sciences. CME. 2017; Vol 48(2), p207-216.

Medscape Physician Compensation Report 2016. www.medscape.com/features/slideshow/compensation/2016/public/overview

Phillips KA, Ospina NS. Physicians interrupting patients. JAMA. 2017: 318(1):93-94. doi:10.1001/jama.2017.6493.

Platt R: Two essays on the practice of medicine. Manchester University Medical School Gazette. 1947; 27:139-145.

National Ambulatory Medical Survey: 2010 Summary Tables. www.cdc.gov/nchs/data/ahcd/namcs_summary/2010_namcs_web_tables.pdf

Montague E, Asan O. Dynamic modeling of patient and physician eye gaze to understand the effects of electronic health records on doctor-patient communication and attention. Int J Med Inform. 2014; Vol 83 (3): Pages 225-234.

Ospina NS, Phillips KA, Rodriguez-Gutierrez R, Castaneda-Guarderas A, Gionfriddo M, Branda M, Montori VM. Eliciting the Patient's Agenda-Secondary Analysis of Recorded Clinical Encounters. Journal of General Internal Medicine. 2019; 34(1): 36-40.

Peterson MC, Holbrook JK, Von Hales D, Smith NL, Staker LV. Contributions of the history, physical examination, and laboratory investigation in making medical diagnoses. Wet J Med. 1992; 156(2):163-5.

Ranjan P, Kumari A, Chakrawarty A. How can Doctors Improve their Communication Skills? J Clin Diagn Res. 2015; 9(3): JE01-JE04.

Rhoades DR, McFarland KF, Finch WH, Johnson AO. Speaking and interruptions during primary care office visits. Fam Med. 2001; 33(7):528-32.

Roter D. The patient-physician relationship and its implications for malpractice litigation. J Health Care Law Policy. 2006; 9304-314.

Stewart MA. Effective physician-patient communication and health outcomes: a review. CMAJ. 1995; 152(9):1423-33.

Tonge JR et al. Communication skills for patient-centered care. J Bone Joint Surg. 2005, 652-658.

Tsukamoto T, Ohira Y, Noda K, Takada T, Ikusaka M. The contribution of the medical history for the diagnosis of simulated cases by medical students. International Journal Med Edu. 2012; 3:78-82.

Weger H, Bell G, Minei E, Robinson, M. The Relative Effectiveness of Active Listening in Initial Interactions. International J Listening. 2014; Vol 28(1).

WHO website. "Collaborative Practice." https://hsc.unm.edu/ipe/resources/who.html.

Young RA, Burge SK, Kumar KA, Wilson JM, Ortiz DF. A Time-Motion Study of Primary Care Physicians' Work in the Electronic Health Record Era. Fam Med. 2018; 50(2):91-99.

Chapter 9: Room for Empathy

Hojat M, Gonnella J, Nasca T, Mangione S, Vergare M, Magee M. Physician Empathy: Definition, Components, Measurement, and Relationship to Gender and Specialty. Am Journ Psychiatry. 2002. https://doi.org/10.1176/appi.ajp.159.9.1563.

Buber M. (1958). I and Thou, translated by Ronald Gregor Smith. New York. Charles Scribner's Sons.

Blumgart HL. Caring for the Patient. N Engl J Med. 1964; 270:449-56

Coulehan JL, Platt FW, Egener B, Frankel R, Lin Ct, Lown B, Salazar WH. "Let Me See If I Have This Right." Words that Help Build Empathy. Annals Intern Med. 2001; 135(3):221-7.

Figley CR. Compassion fatigue: toward a new understanding of caring. In:

Halpern J. What is Clinical Empathy? J Gen Intern Med. 2003; 18(8): 670-674.

Hudnall Stamm B, editor. (1995). Secondary traumatic stress: self-care issues for clinicians, researchers, and educators. Lutherville, MD: Sidran Press

Morse D, Edwardsen EA, Gordon HS. Missed Opportunities for Interval Empathy in Lung Cancer Communication. Arch Intern Med. 2008; 168(17):1853-1858.

Murphy-Shigematsu, S. I See You, I am Here: The Secret to Heartfelt Communication. www.lionsroar.com. June 2, 2021.

Philipp R, Philipp E, Thorne P. The importance of intuition in the occupational clinical consultation. Occup Med. 1999; 49(1): 37-41.

Scott JG, Scott RG, Miller WL, Stange KC, Crabtree BF. Healing relationships and the existential philosophy of Martin Buber. Philos Ethics Humanit Med. 2009; 4:11.

Sturzu L, Lala A, Bisch M, Guitter M, Dobre D, Schwan R. Empathy and Burnout – A Cross-Sectional Study Among Mental Healthcare Providers in France. J Med Life. 2019; 12(1):21-29.

Takeghani F, Ashouri E, Saburi M. Empathy, Burnout, Demographic Variable, and their Relationships in Oncology Nurses. Iran J Nurs Midwifery Res. 2017; 22(1): 41-45.

Thirioux B, Birault F, Jaafari M. Empathy is a Protective Factor of Burnout in Physicians: New Neuro-Phenomological Hypotheses Regarding Empathy and Sympathy in Care Relationship. Front Psychol. 2016; 7:763.

Zenasni F, Boojum Em Woerner A, Sultan A. Burnout and empathy in primary care: three hypotheses. Br J Gen Pract. 2012; 62(600): 346-347.

Chapter 10: On Physician Burnout and Creating Resilience

Cordova M, Gimmler C, Osterberg L. Foster Well-being Through the Career Trajectory: A Developmental Model of Physician Resilience Training. Mayo Clin Proc. 2020; 95(12): 2719-2733.

Diekelmann S, Born J. The memory function of sleep. Nat Rev Neurosci. 2010; 11(2);114-26. doi: 10.1038/nrn2762.

Drummond D. Physician Burnout: Its Origin, Symptoms, and Five Main Causes. Fam Pract Management. 2015; 22(5): 42-47. www.aafp.org/fpm.

Dyrbye L, Shanafelt T, Sinksy C, et al. Burnout among Health Care Professionals: A call to explore and address this underrecognized threat to safe, high-quality care. NAM.edu/Perspectives. 2017. pp 1-11.

Dyrbye LN, West CP, Satele D, et al. Burnout among U.S. medical students, residents, and early career physicians relative to the general U.S. population. Acad Med. 2014; 89(3): 443-451.

Epstein RM, Krasner MS. Physician resilience: what it means, why it matters, and how to promote it. Acad Med. 2013; 88(3): 301-3.

Gabel S. Demoralization in health professional practice: development, amelioration, and implications for continuing education. J Contin Educ Health Prof. 2013; 33(2):118-26.

Galanis P, et al. Nurses' burnout and associated risk factors during the COVID-19 pandemic: A systematic review and meta-analysis. J Adv Nurs. 2021; 77(8):3286-3302. doi: 10.111/Jan. 14839.Epub 2021 Mar 25.

Goitein L, O'Malley PG, Redberg RF. Physician Work Environment and Well-being. A Call for Papers. JAMA Internal Medicine. 2017; 177(2): 164-165. doi: 10.1001/jamainternmed.2016.7688.

Hartzbrand P, Groopman J. Physician Burnout, Interrupted. New England Journ Med. 2020; 382:2485-2487.

Jordan J, et al. Impact of a Mentorship Program on Medical Student Burnout. AEM Educ Train.2019; 3(3): 218-225. doi: 10.1002/aet2.10354.

Jourkes E, et al. Time Spent on Dedicated Patient Care and Documentation Tasks Before and After the Introduction of a Structured and Standardized Electronic Health Record. Appl Clin Inform. 2018; 9(1): 45-53. doi: 10.1055/s-0037-1615747.

Keegan DW. How to Keep Your Income up as RVUs Transition Away. Medscape Perspectives. 2013.

Kolkin J. A Physician's Perspective on Volunteering Overseas… It is Not All about Sharing the Latest Technology. Frontiers in Surgery. 2018; 4(77): 1-5.

Kramer M. Sleep Loss in Resident Physicians: The Cause of Medical Errors? Front Neurol. 2010; 1: 128. doi: 10.3389/fneur.2010.00128.

Krasner M, Epstein R, Beckman H. Association of an Educational Program in Mindful Communication With Burnout, Empathy, and Attitudes Among Primary Care Physicians. JAMA. 2009; 302 (12): 1294-1293. doi:10.1001/jama.2009.1384.

Maslach C., Jackson S. E., Leiter M. P. (1996). MBI: Maslach Burnout Inventory. Sunnyvale, CA: CPP, Incorporated.

Medscape National Physician Burnout, Depression, & Suicide Report 2021. "Death by 1000 cuts." www.medscape.com.

Montero-Marin J, Garcia-Campayo J, Mosquera-Mera D, Lopez del Hoyo Y. A new definition of burnout syndrome based on Farber's proposal. J Occup Med Toxicol. 2009; 4:31.

Ofei-Dodoo S, Scripter C, Kellerman R. Job Satisfaction and Burnout Among Nonclinical Works in a Medical Education Center. Fam Med. 2018; 50(3): 223-227. doi: 10.22454/FamMed.2018.473306.

Peckman C. Medscape Lifestyle Report 2017: race and ethnicity, bias, and burnout. https://www.medscape.com/features/slideshow/lifestyle/2017/overview. Published January 11, 2017. Accessed December 6, 2017.

Platz J, Hyman N. Mentorship. Clin Colon Rectal Surg. 2013; 26(4): 218-223. doi: 10.1055/s-0033-1356720.

Reddy A, Pollack CE, Asch DA, Canamucio A, Werner RM. The Effect of Primary Care Provider Turnover on Patient Experience of Care and Ambulatory Quality of Care. JAMA Intern Med. 2015; 175 (7): 1157-62.

Shanafelt T, Schein E, Minor L, Trockel M, Schein P, Kirch D. Healing the Professional Culture of Medicine. Mayo Clinic Proceedings. 2019; (8):1556-1566

Shanafelt T, Goh J, Sinksy C. The Business Case for Investing in Physician Well-being. JAMA Intern Med. 2017; 177(12):1826-1832.

Shirom A, Nurel N, Vinokur A. Work Hours and Caseload as Predictors of Physician Burnout: The Mediating Effects by Perceived Workload and Autonomy. Applied Psychology: An International Review. 2010; 59(4). 539-565.

Sinsky C, Colligan L, Li L, Prgomet M, Reynolds S. Allocation of Physician Time in Ambulatory Practice: A Time and Motion Study in 4 Specialties. Ann Intern Med. 2016; 165(11): 753-760. https://doi.org/10.7326/M16-0961. Epub 2016 Sep 6.

Sullivan D, et al. Comparison of Nurse Burnout, Before and During the COVID-19 Pandemic. Nurs Clin North Am. 2022; 57(1): 79-99.
Teisberg E et al. Defining and Implementing Value-Based Health Care: A Strategic Framework. Acad Med. 2020; 95(5): 682-685. doi: 10.1097/ACM.0000000000003122.

Tsevat J, Moriates C. Value-Based Health Care Meets Cost-Effectiveness Analysis. Annals of Internal Medicine. 2018. Vol 169(5): 329-332. https://doi.org/10.7236/M18-0342.

Wallace S, Teisberg EO. Measuring what matters: Connecting excellence, professionalism, and empathy. Brain Inj Prof. 2016; 12: 12-15.

WHO & UNICEF 2017 Progress on Drinking Water, Sanitation and Hygiene: 2017 Update and SDG Baselines.

UNICEF. Collecting water is often a colossal waste of time for women and girls. August 29, 2016. UNICEF webpage.

UNICEF. Diarrhoea remains a leading killer of young children, despite the availability of a simple treatment solution. UNICEF webpage.

Van der Riet P, et al. The effectiveness of mindfulness meditation for nurses and nursing students: An integrated literature review. Nurse Educ Today. 2018; 65:201-211. doi: 10.1016/j.nedt.2018.03.018. Epub 2018 Mar 24.

Venegas CL, Nkangu MN, Duffy MC, Fergusson D, Spilg EG. Interventions to improve resilience in physicians who have completed training: A systemic review. PLoS One 2019; 14(1): e0210512.

West CP, Dyrbye LN, et al. Intervention to Promote Physician Well-being, Job Satisfaction, and Professionalism: A Randomized Clinical Trial. JAMA Internal Medicine. 2014; Vol 174, Number 4: 528-532.

Farber, BA. Burnout in psychotherapist: incidence, types, and trends. Psychother. Private Pract. 1990; 8, 35–44. doi: 10.1300/J294v08n01_07

Schein, EH. (2010). *Organizational Culture and Leadership.* Jossey-Bass.

Chapter 11: Concluding Remarks

Cheesman N. Doctors as teachers. BMJ. 2009; 339:b1551. doi: org/10.1136/bmj.b1551.

Felitti V, et al. Relationship of Childhood Abuse and Household Dysfunction to Many of the Leading Causes of Death in Adults. The Adverse Childhood Experiences (ACE) Study. Am J of Prev Med. 1998; Vol 14(4):245-382.

Shin L. What is the Average Medical School Debt? Website: www.thebalance.com. 2021.

Wang J et al. Is a career in medicine the right choice? The impact of a physician shadowing
program on undergraduate premedical students. Acad Med. 2015; 90(5): 629-33.
doi: 10.1097/ACM.0000000000000615.

Ward M. "The Taoist Parable of the Stonecutter: How to find happiness by letting go." 2020.
www.medium.com

APPENDIX 1

Ways to Reduce Bias in the Clinic: Clinicians

1. Start with the history and physical and end with the history and physical. Start with actively listening to the patient without interrupting until they have described the narrative, which usually takes a few minutes. Active listening requires eye contact, nodding, verbal confirmation, and summarizing back. Smartphone checks, eyes fixed on the keyboard, and frequent patient interruptions inhibit active listening. The median time a doctor interrupts a patient explaining their symptoms is eleven seconds.

If anything is unclear after the first assessment, go back to the patient and ask more questions. Sometimes their concerns may drive the words they choose to describe the symptoms. If you sense that this is biasing them, ask the patient what they think or fear they may have? A proper physical examination can help confirm the diagnosis, rule out other concerns, and gauge the need for further testing.

2. If there is concern that the diagnosis is in question, circle back to the patient, discuss the developing history, and think about other causes. Physicians benefit from thinking of at least two or three possibilities while avoiding system 1 decisions that jump to a solution or explain the problem backward. Let the symptoms guide the differential, not the other way around.

3. Most patient concerns require a formal visit. It can sometimes be challenging to address patient calls during a busy day in the clinic. Unfortunately, patients may truncate their concerns during a phone call, limiting their history and preventing careful assessment. Aside from answering basic questions on the phone, telemedicine or clinic visit provides the best setting to address complex concerns.

4. Describe to the patient what you think is the next step to evaluate the concern. A doctor should consider the choice of words for a statement, as it might lead to a framing bias. There is no difference between conditions associated with a 96% survivor rate and 4% mortality rate, but they emphasize the data differently.

APPENDIX 2

Ways to Reduce Bias in the Clinic: Patients

1. Before a visit, write out the sequence of events. An accurate historical account is usually more helpful than listing signs and symptoms. Timing can help a provider determine a pattern in how a process develops. As a volunteer in the Gambia, I worked alongside an interpreter who routinely asked patients for a complete review of symptoms. Patients would invariably say "yes" to many of the symptoms. I learned that they understood the questions as "in some time of your life." You can imagine how little it helped to clarify the current issues.

2. Prepare a list of concerns and questions for a problem-focused visit in advance. Some things can await a routine follow-up or a complete physical examination. I usually recommend two concerns and two additional questions for a twenty-minute visit.

3. Avoid using a diagnosis based on your description of the symptoms. Instead of "doctor, I have pneumonia," try "Doctor, I have a cough and sore throat" and describe the factors that worsen or relieve it.

4. Discuss any deeper concerns with the clinician after objectively stating the symptoms. Clinicians may weigh their concerns and discuss potential causes and plans for addressing the condition.

Sometimes the combination of events with underlying fears can jumble the narrative and distort the significance of the information.

5. Go through the plan with the physician and develop contingency steps. One study found that patients recalled only forty-nine percent of decisions and plans without prompting (Laws, 2018). By discussing these plans with the doctor, the patient may further clarify any uncertainties. Shared and informed decision-making ensures greater satisfaction and adherence to the agreed-upon recommendations.

6. Schedule a follow-up in one to two months on the same day as the current visit. A follow-up visit ensures that the problem is revisited and keeps the issue at the forefront.

Case Index

Case	Title	Chapter	Theme
1	History Speaks for Itself	3	Anchoring Bias
2	The Infection Masquerade	3	Anchoring Bias, Confirmation Bias
3	Pneumonia in the Time of COVID-19	3	Availability Heuristic
4	It was in the Decimal Point	4	Prescribing Error
5	Postoperative Foot Pain	4	False Attribution Error
6	Postoperative Increased WBC	4	Surgical Miscount Error
7	Treating to Cover the Bases	4	Misattribution and Diagnostic Delay
8	Just Need a Refill of My Prescriptions	5	Medication Use for Behaviors
9	Multiple Episodes of Pneumonia	5	Collaborative Care for Diagnosis
10	Having the Heart to Prescribe	5	Primary care and Specialist Roles
11	Mononucleosis Syndrome	6	Approaching a Difficult Diagnosis
12	TB or not TB?	6	Approaching a Difficult Diagnosis
13	Blood Breakdown after a SCT	6	Approaching a Difficult Diagnosis
14	"I Thought I Saw Blood."	6	Sudden Changes Upper GI Bleed
15	The Last Bleed	6	Sudden Changes Variceal Bleed

Endnotes

1 Translation by W.H.S. Jones.

Chapter 2: The Evolution of the Modern Health Paradigm

2 The sense of smell, or *fetor*, can be a source of information even today. Humans can train their companions to be technicians. A 2006 study showed how accurately dogs can detect certain cancers using their noses; their sense of smell is 10,000 more accurate than humans (McCulloch M, 2006.)

3 Modern-day technology has revealed the limits of Koch's postulates which were developed in 1884. Some bacteria are not able to grow in culture and require molecular testing. Prions are infectious proteins that cause disease.

Chapter 3: Transcending Bias in Clinical Decision-Making

4 A "soft call" is a determination that may represent an early finding of a disease or be a less significant or even normal finding.

5 These changes sometimes mean there is smoldering inflammation within the lung tissue.

6 RT-PCR, reverse transcriptase polymerase chain reaction, a test used to detect genetic information from a pathogen. For COVID-19, the greatest sensitivity is seen with sputum and bronchial washings.

7 Sensitivity is the likelihood of a test to detect a disease when it is present (True Positive). Specificity is the likelihood to not detect a disease when it is not present (True Negative). A low specificity test means that it is unable to exclude other causes for the positive result.

8 The reader can test their implicit bias, an unconscious favoritism or prejudice toward one group, by referring to the Harvard Implicit bias test at https://implicit.harvard.edu/implicit/

9 In medical parlance, the verb "presents" describes the concerns for which a patient seeks care. The noun "presentation" describes the clinical features of a condition.

10 CYA, is an acronym for "Cover Your Ass."

11 Like the horse and hoof sounds heuristic is Occam's razor, a concept that approaches an explanation with the smallest number of assumptions. Imagine a tree falling after a rainstorm. One assumes from evaluating it that it was struck by lightning, rather than a laser beam from an alien spaceship. Although, a simple solution may be correct for most conditions, it is not always.

12 Residents often work together in teams. Training with other students and residents can be instrumental in improving a future doctor's practice style and clinical knowledge base.

Chapter 4: On Medical Errors

13 In 2013, 611,105 people died from heart disease and 584,881 died from cancer. More people die of medical errors (250,000) than the next leading cause of death, chronic respiratory disease (149,205).

14 Adult failure to thrive is often used as a general description for a constellation of symptoms, including physical inactivity, weight loss, and decreased appetite, which are related to multiple potential causes.

15 Tachycardia means fast heart rate (>100 beats per minute). Atrial fibrillation means when the upper chamber of the heart beats erratically, affecting regular flow.

16 Considering an infection such as neurocysticercosis warrants a search for risk factors. There were several case reports in the Orthodox Jewish community in New York City, none of whom had ingested pork— the usual route of entry. It turned out that the patients had acquired the infection from household workers or food handlers who had emigrated from countries where Taenia solium infections are prevalent (Schantz, 1992).

18 Doctors often order bloodwork, because they are less invasive and may lead toward a diagnosis. However, more is not always better. When they are positive, they sometimes lead to more testing or inappropriate treatments. One of my infectious diseases attendings as a fellow once told me that ordering a test is like picking your nose in public.

18 A sample of cerebrospinal fluid is sent for myelin basic protein (MBP), which is found after brain injury, including in multiple sclerosis.

19 Osler is known for stating "the chief function of a consultant is to do a rectal exam."

20 Lyme disease is diagnosed with two-step testing: a Lyme antibody titer with a confirmatory Western blot, which is a test that looks at specific antibodies based on size. Five or more specific bands need to be present to diagnose Lyme disease.

Chapter 5: Generalist and Specialist: Putting the Patient as the Priority

21 The term "primary care" refers to internal medicine, family medicine, and pediatrics.

22 There are multiple factors behind why specialists usually receive more income than generalists. A few of the reasons include the experience gained in additional training, specialists get reimbursed higher than generalists, and that many specialists perform procedures.

23 Statins are a group of lipid medications, known as HMG-CoA-reductase inhibitors, which inhibit cholesterol synthesis in the body, lowering LDL.

24 Infectious diseases in immunocompromised patients with ground-glass changes on CT scan include P*neumocystis jirovecii* pneumonitis or CMV pneumonitis.

25 Deprescribing should always be initiated while under the direct supervision of a physician.

26 A brown bag review (BBR) offers an opportunity to review medications and their indications, as well as provide structured medication counseling (Jaeger, 2015).

27 EGD means esophagogastroduodenoscopy. It is a specialized fiberoptic scope to visualize the esophagus, stomach, and duodenum.

Chapter 6: On the Difficult Diagnosis and Sudden Health Changes

28 Biomedical model separates the physical and the psychological.

29 Somatic (adj), or somaticize (verb), of or pertaining to the body.

30 Watchful waiting means to monitoring closely for the development of symptoms and a disease process.

31 An estimated $200 billion yearly is spent on unnecessary tests and treatments. As many as 25% of ordered laboratory tests are unnecessary, including repeated and inappropriate tests. Not only are there financial implications, but an increased risk of improper diagnosis from false-positive tests an added stress to the patient (Patel, 2019; Terhune, 2017).

32 This is a rapid test known as the heterophile antibody which has a sensitivity of 85% and specificity of 100% for Epstein Barr Virus.

33 Typhoidal presentation as in *Salmonella typhi* and *paratyphi*, the causes of typhoid fever.

34 The bacillus that causes tuberculosis *Mycobacterium tuberculosis* stains with an acid-fast technique that picks up mycolic acids, fatty acids in the cell wall of the bacterium.

35 The initial therapy for tuberculosis is Rifampin, Isoniazid, Pyrazinamide, and Ethambutol (RIPE). Pyridoxine (Vitamin B6) is added as well to counter isonazid's effect on peripheral nerves.

36 Hem/Onc is short for Hematology/Oncology, a specialty in cancer and blood disorders.

37 The medical term for blood breakdown is hemolysis.

38 This is referred to as "functional asplenia."

39 The species name "canimorsus" is "dog bite" in Latin.

40 Infection can be assessed indirectly with antibody titers and directly with a test known as Polymerase Chain Reaction (PCR), to look for genetic material of the pathogen.

41 Infection can be assessed indirectly with antibody titers and directly with a test known as Polymerase Chain Reaction (PCR), to look for genetic material of the pathogen.

42 The sentence highlights a common dilemma that labs and insurances plans must balance: a test with greater accuracy versus cost-containment strategies.

43 An issue that came up with this case was how does one approach a difference of opinion between colleagues and supervisors. How does one best advocate for a patient, while not alienating a fellow doctor or supervising physician? In this case, one option may have included seeing the patient together and discussing the plan collaboratively.

44 A common cause of blood seen in vomitus are Mallory-Weiss tears, which are small tears in the lower esophagus. Although they rarely can lead to severe bleeding, they usually do not and heal on their own.

45 A state of confusion from cirrhosis is known as hepatic encephalopathy. The condition results from decompensated liver disease, often in the setting of an acute precipitating factor, such as GI bleeding.

46 An Interventionalist is a physician that performs specialized procedures. For stroke management, a radiologist, neurologist, and neurosurgeon can train several years to become neurointerventionalists.

47 Asystole carries a mortality rate of 90% out of the hospital (Engdahl, 2000).

48 Deep venous thrombosis (DVT), or a blood clot in a larger vein.

Chapter 7: The Difficult Encounter

49 Malingering is the fabrication or exaggeration of a behavior with the intent to receive medications, certification, or avoid work.

50 Aberrant behavior is any behavior considered consistent with misuse, diversion, or substance use disorder.

51 One of my most challenging experiences with trust is discussed in Case 19.

52 This term is used for a person who actively seeks a physician, often multiple at one time, to prescribe them medications or provide an opinion, for which they are looking.

53 The phrases are some examples that I received in patients that were later determined to be at a considerable risk of opiate dependence. While the communication may seem that the prescribing doctor was not sensitive to the patient's pain, opiate management is under the management and discretion of the doctor. Studies show that increasing doses of pain medications seldom achieve any improvements in quality of life.

54 Select patients, including those with cancer-related pain, may have an improvement in their quality of life from opiate therapy. Doctors need to weigh the risks and benefits of opiates in selecting patients, particularly for long-term therapy.

55 After temperature, pulse, heart rate, and respiratory rate.

56 Opiates affect other neurotransmitters and the production of hormones. They also decrease production of cortisol in the adrenal glands.

57 The cardinal signs of inflammation are rubor, calor, dolor, tumor, and function laesa. These correspond to redness, warmth, pain, swelling, and loss of function, respectively.

58 Feigning a pain or a disorder for secondary gain.

Chapter 8: On Listening, Communication, and Collaboration

59 The term "agenda" relates to the reason that prompted a patient to schedule an appointment.

60 Color and odor are not reliable indicators of urinary tract infection. Increased confusion may be caused by to sundowning, or late-day confusion in someone living with dementia, medication side effects, and acute health changes such as infections.

Chapter 10: On Burnout and Creating Resilience

61 Call or being "on call" during residency means carrying a pager and being available at the hospital for patient admissions and/or being available to the nurses for other patient concerns in the hospital.

62 From the Myth of Sisyphus. Zeus punished him eternally to roll a boulder up a hill only for it to roll back down.

63 Doctor's visits are billed to insurance companies for reimbursements. A practice's compensation for each visit depends on its difficulty level. Coding higher, or up-coding, means that a provider records a higher level of complexity for a visit. Most of the time, higher codes accurately reflect the work. However, the charts need to be more complete to justify them.

64 Refer to online MBI resources, such as monkey puzzle's Burnout Self-Test Maslach Burnout Inventory (MBI).

65 In 1984, Libby Zion reported to New York Hospital ER with a fever and earache. She had a tooth extraction and received oxycodone. She developed respiratory arrest and was unable to be saved. She was found to have cocaine in nasal samples and toxicologic studies.

66 For more information on these groups and a toolkit for starting your own group, refer to Commensality Groups | WellMD & WellPhD | Stanford Medicine.

67 About 525,000 children a year, or 1,400 children each day, die from gastrointestinal diseases (UNICEF).

Chapter 11: Closing Remarks

68 The average medical school debt is approximately $207,000 (Shinn, 2021).

Certificate of Completion

This is to certify that

____

*has successfully completed **4 hours** of doctor shadowing by reading*

Becoming Tomorrow's Doctor

Christopher M. Cirino, DO, MPH

Date of Completion

Awarded by

About the Author

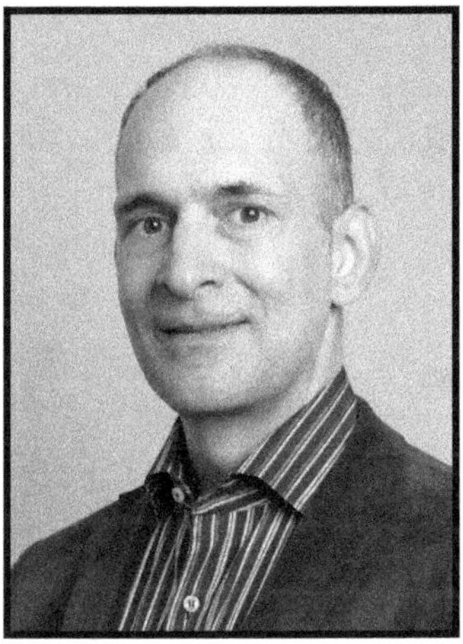

Christopher M. Cirino, DO, MPH, is a board-certified physician in internal medicine and infectious diseases. He endeavors to explore solutions to the health care crisis and the burden of chronic disease. Dr. Cirino's view of health centers on the root cause of disease. Drawing from the tenets of Dr. Andrew Taylor Still, he strives to guide his patients to find ways to heal from illness and reawaken their health.

He is the founder of Your Health Forum, an online medical reference that bridges wellness and neuroscience concepts. He holds seminars in the community and online that cover areas including infectious diseases, physician burnout, career advice, mindfulness, and understanding behavior's role in health.

Dr. Cirino is a speaker, health coach, and lifelong learner. He received his undergraduate degree in Microbiology from Miami University of Ohio in 1994. He earned his Doctor of Osteopathic Medicine (D.O.) at the Ohio University Heritage College of Osteopathic Medicine in 1998. Cirino participated in residency training at the George Washington University Medical Center from 1999 to 2002. At GWUMC, he trained in his infectious disease fellowship from 2004 to 2006 and completed his MPH at the GW Milken Institute School of Public Health.

Author of four children's books, Dr. Cirino's goal is to get the message of health empowerment out to people of all ages. He is a proud father of three boys, ages 15, 13, and 10, and lives in Portland, Oregon. Follow him on yourhealthforumbydrcirino.org and Tomorrowsdoc.com

Index

A

B

C

D

U

V

W

Y

www.ingramcontent.com/pod-product-compliance
Lightning Source LLC
LaVergne TN
LVHW020412220926
848484LV00016B/2543/J